AIDS Alibis

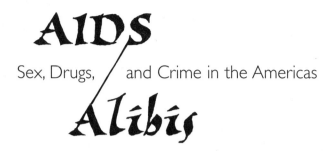

AIDS

Sex, Drugs, and Crime in the Americas

Alibis

STEPHANIE C. KANE

TEMPLE UNIVERSITY PRESS

Philadelphia

Temple University Press, Philadelphia 19122
Copyright © 1998 by Temple University
All rights reserved
Published 1998
Printed in the United States of America

Text design by Gary Gore

∞The paper used in this publication meets the requirements of American National Standard for Information Sciences—Performance of Paper for Printed Library Materials, ANSI Z39.48-1984.

Library of Congress Cataloging-in-Publication Data

Kane, Stephanie C., 1951–
    AIDS alibis : sex, drugs, and crime in the Americas / Stephanie C. Kane.
        p.   cm.
    Includes bibliographical references and index.
    ISBN 1-56639-627-1 (cl. : alk. paper). — ISBN 1-56639-628-x (pbk. alk. paper)
    1. AIDS (Disease)—Social aspects—America.   I. Title.
RA644.A25K364   1998
362.1′969792′00973—dc21   97-49094
                                                                      CIP

To Claudia
sister, artist, healer, friend

/ Contents

/ Acknowledgments

Thanks to the people whose voices give life to this book.

Thanks to the institutions that provided funding for research and writing: the Wenner Gren Foundation for Anthropological Research; Indiana University; the Rockefeller Foundation and the State University of New York at Buffalo; Fulbright Hays and the Council for the International Exchange of Scholars; and the National Institute of Drug Abuse (National AIDS Demonstration Research Grant 5R-18-DAO-5285).

Thanks to those who gave support and inspiration: Stephen Arzu, Doris Braendel, Margaret Castillo, Charlie and Gerald Chavanne, Ellen Dwyer, Rachel Emmer, Bibbi Essama, Isabel Goldberg, Pauline Greenhill, Carol Greenhouse, Sinia Harper, Gilbert Herdt, Michael Howe, Wendell Johnson, John Junson, Hilary Kahn, B. David Kane, Harriet Klein, George Lewis, Shirley Lindenbaum, Liz Locke, Theresa Mason, Claudia Kane Michler, Dana Nicholas, Phil Parnell, Leon Pettiway, Claude Rhodes, Oscar Tanner, and Jay Wilkerson.

Finally, I toast Eli Goitein for his original drawings. And for creative energy beyond the call of friendship, thanks to C. Jason Dotson, freelance criminologist and teacher-poet.

1 / Introduction

A Disease to Live With, a War to Leave Behind

Acquired Immune Deficiency Syndrome (AIDS) is one of a host of threats to our species. Toxicity is an everyday immune event, so close to home that fluids are fighting flesh inside our bodies. Future archaeologists will date baby boomers by the radioactive strontium in their bones. We have immune disease and autoimmune disease; we have homicide and suicide; we have drug war and drug addiction. We are being trained to accept wars against ourselves, wars that kill us but that we agree are in our own best interest. If justice and reason prevailed, we could control all this. We have the scientific understanding and the technology to stop war, pollution, and AIDS. But we ride down the old rutted paths, now sleek with advances in weapons technology, testifying to our good intentions all the way. At times we completely lose our sense of purpose, but we continue to maintain our stock of rationales, our alibis.

My sense of our predicament reminds me of a night back in 1977. I was nearing the Strait of Cortez just past the tip of Cuba on a sailboat named *Meriah*. The sky was dark and clear, the sea's currents rushing with the purpose of a river. Like a grasshopper before a line of elephants, the thirty-eight-foot *Meriah* was about to cross a lane of freighters heading toward the Panama Canal. At the rudder I learned that if we got too near, even if someone on board the freighter happened to be on deck to see us, there would be nothing that person could do to prevent a wreck. The reason that the freighter couldn't stop, even with human intervention, was inertia.

I believe that citizens of the Americas are on a collision course with misguided government policies that, like the freighter relentlessly moving across the sea, have great weight and are blind to human misery. It seems such policies can be impeded only with superhuman effort. That starry night two decades ago, I was not completely powerless. I made sure to steer and keep a sharp eye out. A beautiful dawn was my reward. But the *Meriah* never made it down the Yucatan coast as planned. In a vain attempt to seek calm waters for the night, we ran aground on a reef at the mouth of Bahia del Espiritu Santo. To this day I suppose, *Meriah* lies stripped bare at the bottom, an offering to the ancestors of the Mayans who rescued us before returning to harvest her bounty, leaving their knife in the masthead, a token.

The fascinating thing about the shipwreck is that it didn't have to happen. Everyone around there knows that even locals don't try to find their way into the small openings of barrier reefs in the dark. After this experience, I have always tried to get a sense of the lay of the land, a sense of "what everyone around here knows." The AIDS epidemic became a focus of study and activism during a good portion of my travel and research since 1988.[1] This book tells of these experiences through the stories of people I met, observed, or read about. I combine types of knowledge that carry different kinds of truth-value: Myths tell the truth about theory but may not be useful on a daily basis; statistics weight the truth with a certain kind of authority and insight; life histories render substance and spirit; and ethnographic description reveals social structures and processes. Then there are the lies and the alibis. I'm especially interested in alibis, how we end up using the same old tired excuses all the time, about why we were doing what we were doing when we should have been playing safe, about why our minds were elsewhere when some rebel pieces of genetic material with lipid-protein coats (that is, HIV)[2] got the better of us.

Since 1983, we've had scientific knowledge regarding the identity of the virus and its modes of transmission, as well as the technology to test for antibody evidence of its presence in blood. Basically, this knowledge clued us in to the fact that we all have to be extra careful about exchanging our body fluids. Since the beginning of culture as we know it, there have been elaborate cultural constraints on body fluids, and the new limitations the virus has imposed are well within the scope of human capability. The aim of prevention education (which remains the only way to avoid infection once the virus has entered a region) is to disseminate scientific knowledge about the virus in ways that address the diversity of relevant actions in which humans may engage (that is, appropriate to different types of "risk behaviors") and in ways that help individuals and institutions make necessary adjustments in their everyday lives (that is, to achieve "risk reduction" in different cultural contexts). Because HIV has an average latency period of ten years, during which infection is invisible to the naked eye (and people are most infectious right after they are infected themselves, even before the antibody test can work), it is essential that people trust scientific knowledge in order for prevention to be successful.

While seemingly simple, the requirement of being extra careful about one's body fluids is actually inordinately difficult for individuals and institutions, particularly when it conflicts with other priorities like pleasure-seeking and war. Despite all the millions that the U.S. government has spent on prevention education, it seems unlikely that it is serious about ending the pandemic. Indeed, prevention programs often seem like alibis set up to make it appear that representatives of the people care about their health and well-being. But if they really do care, then they would not perpetuate the biggest alibi in the Americas today: the U.S. war on drugs. The drug war purportedly protects citizens from being exposed to harmful substances. But only certain harmful substances are illegal, and it seems that everyone who wants those substances can get them anyway.

Rather than protecting citizens, the drug war has recoded addiction, turning a social and medical problem into criminal justice business. The drug war gives the government, the police, and the military a ready alibi for arbitrary and racist murders and imprisonments;[3] it sucks up our resources to enrich companies that sell weaponry, transport, and surveillance equipment to be used against us; it takes the resources we need for schools and hospitals and uses it to build prisons. "For the good of the people" provides a weak excuse for transferring more power to the police.

The simultaneous involvement of government in both the drug war and AIDS prevention twists the claims of prevention. Instead of helping people to change their lives for the better, AIDS prevention becomes part of the panic logic that characterizes our culture and erotic economy. Panic logic binds the fears and anxieties we have about fatal disease to the ordered elements of reason. The creation of panic logic conveys a sense of control over negative emotions and events, but its effects are paradoxical. The primary tendency of panic logic is to produce and multiply the very phenomena it seeks to control.[4] Drug warfare and AIDS prevention cannot remain distinct. Simultaneous government efforts in two directions produce law and policy founded on panic logic; for example, the persistence of criminal sanctions that make it a crime to possess or distribute clean needles; the prosecution of drug-addicted pregnant women for poisoning their fetuses; the mandatory testing and incarceration of HIV-positive women prostitutes.[5] AIDS prevention can itself be used as an alibi for consolidating political and economic interests around archaic moral pretenses, such as perverted purveyors of abstinence-only sex education for sexually active youth or the closure of sex-related businesses to hasten the Disneyfication of New York City's Times Square (Dangerous Bedfellows 1996).[6] The astonishingly cunning design of HIV's mindless virulence, which attacks the complex, specialized system of blood cells that constitute our species' immunity, creates a challenge that continues to stymie scientists searching for a vaccine or cure, contributing to panic.

By identifying the behaviors associated with HIV infection among individuals, the science of epidemiology was crucial in establishing the content of AIDS prevention education. In the United States, the virus first took hold among gay and bisexual men, injecting drug users, and hemophiliacs. The first three social identities have long been marginalized as deviant in contemporary American cultures. As a result, in addition to their usefulness in guiding risk-reduction, epidemiological models of HIV risk lent panic logic a scientific scaffold for containing AIDS dread in clearly demarcated "risk groups" and creating the impression that the epidemic was limited to certain segments of the population. The scientific usefulness of epidemiological categories has been stretched by their symbolic usefulness as a means of regulating panic, to the detriment of prevention efforts for women, youth, heterosexuals, monogamous couples, men who have sex with men but don't identify themselves as homosexual, and so on. In addition, the alliance of epidemiology and panic logic has led to nearly universal overemphasis of individual behavioral change in AIDS prevention campaigns, campaigns that ignore underlying social forces that condition risk and the multiplicities of risk in many people's lives. In this way, panic logic generates research and policy alibis that substitute for serious consideration of the social forces undermining individual attempts to control risk.

As the leading promoter of AIDS prevention programs in the Americas, the U.S. government does fund some decent programs. I can't help thinking though, that if the people who work in the government want to stop AIDS, they would halt the drug war, use the resources to treat people with HIV and drug addiction, alleviate poverty as a cofactor in the epidemic, and launch unflinching educational campaigns. Considering the political forces dominating U.S. policy in the late 1990s, this may sound naive. But trapping ourselves within this parochial frame of reference severely limits the likelihood of finding pragmatic solutions. Why are we not debating the merits of using the enormous resources gleaned from taking possession of money and property earned from the illegal drug trade and using it to finance drug treatment and alternative employment programs for addicted persons? This would reduce demand for drugs and deescalate the war. Instead we allow the police and the military to use these resources to escalate the war, going so far as to allow the Central Intelligence Agency (CIA) to pay drug suppliers (the "kingpins") for intelligence about those whom the CIA labels political enemies (Scott and Marshall 1991).[7] In democratic societies, it should not be considered naive to challenge evil policies of the powerful that operate at the expense of the powerless—even when opposition seems futile.

Thus, the drug war is made to seem like a necessity, a mighty force we must deploy to counter the social deterioration that accompanies addiction. But, despite its dramatic appeal, this has-been warrior myth protects us only in our imaginations. On the contrary, we protect the myth, providing a camouflage of normalcy that entrenches the status quo (cf. Enloe 1989). I became convinced that acquiescence to institutional rationales for not-so-effective research, education, and policy feeds suicidal tendencies in our culture, and so I set forth into the field of discourse created out of the human experience of AIDS, where I confiscate all the alibis I can find.

Crisscrossing the Local-Global Divide

I don't think anybody can really understand how crises of globalization at the end of the twentieth century—of which AIDS is only one—are going to affect us, much less how we can prevent them. In this sense, panic logic is not so much a conscious strategy of the powerful to incite paranoia in the masses as it is a symptom of our times. Jean Baudrillard writes that in these times, AIDS acts as a "superconductive event" in the public imagination: an untimely whirlwind that no longer affects states, individuals, or institutions, but rather entire transversal structures of money, information, and communications. Infection is no longer confined within a given system but can leap from one system to another, producing catastrophe (1993, 37). He writes: "The high degree to which AIDS, terrorism, crack cocaine or computer viruses mobilize the popular imagination should tell us that they are more than anecdotal occurrences in an irrational world. The fact is that they contain within them the whole logic of our system: these events are merely the spectacular expression of that system. . . . This means that it is useless to appeal to some supposed rationality of the system against that system's outgrowths. The vanity of seeking to abolish these extreme phenomena is absolute" (67–68).

I take these reflections seriously, although I am loathe to abandon appeals to rationality. I have designed my methods of analysis and writing to accomplish both rational argument and convey a healthy respect for the uncertain effects of intimacy and catastrophe. In preparation for this world that reaches ever faster for totalities but that admits no totalizing solutions, I represent the field of discourse into which we embark by combining a variety of local cultures and professional disciplines, by questioning the scope of systematicity and admitting the unaccountable aspect of the carnivalesque. AIDS operates as a master signifier within this field of discourse, something difficult to ignore yet eternally transformable as it circulates through electronic and print media, local talk, and academic conferences. The discursive field arises out of more traditional ethnographic field site locations in the United States, Belize, and Guatemala, as well as the cyberspaces that transect these nation-spaces. Those are the regions of human reality in which I apply my activist impulse and out of which I tackle that overwhelming phenomenon called "the system." I introduce you to several characters along the way, real people I have met and others whom I have only read about or have seen on television. Some are fictitious. Each character represents a different social positioning with respect to the epidemic, each embodies (via the text) variant perspectives on, and conceptions of, HIV. More important, each bestows a beautiful gift, which I hope is not lost in translation—the indomitable and creative force of the human spirit.

Weirdly, as an ethnographer-activist-writer, I have come to share some qualities with the virus in the text. We are the only two characters, the virus and I, that appear in all the sites. We share qualities of mobility and adaptability. As I travel through these various sites, my voice changes with the discursive current, the better to communicate; as HIV travels through these landscapes, it mutates within body fluids. I am not sure what this accidental convergence or unconscious mimicry means, although I know from my ethnographic perspective that at least, it is *not* a collaboration.

Informed by studies in criminal justice and feminism, this book fits most securely into the overlapping fields of ethnography and cultural studies, two academic disciplines that can be roughly distinguished by scholars who go someplace called the field to work, where they become participant observers (ethnography),[8] and scholars who stay at home and work from printed texts, television, and film (cultural studies). My explorations stay well within the realm of culture in Raymond Williams's sense of it as "a description of a particular way of life which expresses certain meanings and values, not only in art and learning, but in institutions and ordinary behavior" (1961, 61, in Hall 1993). I analyze the impact of contrasting discourses of public health and law as they affect and are affected by ordinary people's behavior and ideas, accepting the facticity of the knowledge the experts produce while knowing it may be in varying degrees subject to distortions of meaning and value both in the process of discovery and in use. I think through the implications of these dynamic cultural associations in terms of viral transmission: how the genetic templates and psychic shadows of HIV may be moving and transforming in bodies, communities, and transnational networks.

In my research and writing, I seek the emergent aspect of human experience, what Williams has called "structures of feeling"—the give and take of people trying to come to terms with the meaning of the virus within the particular set of relationships that they are living out when I encounter them (1977, 132). I use the expressive elements of restraint, impulse, and tone in their speech as keys to consciousness. Not feelings against thought, writes Williams, but thought as felt and feeling as thought. Pulled together from a diverse set of characters and cultural contexts, I express a sense of how a practical consciousness of the epidemic is absorbed into social experience. Somewhere between the institutionalized logics of public health and law is what "everyone around here knows"—and that, I believe, is the best discursive space to look to understand how humanity participates in the progression of this disease, how we are implicated in our own fatality.

Among the conversations and stories I collected are some outrageous images of AIDS (such as monkey blood, whores' needles, viral weaponry, state conspiracy). Extreme and ostentatious, even when they are true, they are clearly not meant to contribute to empirical generalization. However, they are socially symbolic acts that can through interpretation provide keys to the political unconscious, the struggles for power taking place in and through the language and imagery of our psyches. By analyzing the texts that convey extreme images in a series of wider horizons, as Fredric Jameson suggests, they become more than talk about AIDS (1981, 75–76). The first horizon involves the personal and local meanings of particular events and relationships. Expanding textual analysis to the level of society lends insight into the struggles for life, liberty, and the pursuit of happiness of persons aligning with and against each other along lines of class, gender, race, nation, and profession. At its most expansive, textual analysis can speak to the changing destiny of our species.

My task is to bend semiotics to activism. I read through the alibis that obscure the collective messages embedded within them, searching for the historical forces shaping that which we take for granted as natural (Barthes 1972, 128–29). I juxtapose conversations, stories, and statistics from sources in distinct locales and media, connecting them rhetorically with my voice engaging others in dialogue about AIDS. By making use of this master signifier, I hope to convey a sense of how different people and cultures around the world are struggling to come to terms with an event of global proportions. The juxtaposition of stories by and about people who don't know each other, who may not speak the same language or practice the same ritual, inevitably appears artificial. But the virus is, after all, passing among persons who are unknown to each other and whose social and geographic realities may be quite distant. This technique of analysis and writing is motivated by an urge to understand how a region within the larger global system is resonating with the news of AIDS. I have no particular commitment to an aesthetic of fragmentation, but I sense that whatever the global system is, it is composed of technological and market-linked subsystems that may be otherwise unrelated.[9]

In sum, this book is an experiment in conceptualizing the intercontinental dimensions of the AIDS pandemic. Startling particularities of experience prod hypnotic generalities, exerting effects that can be read as evidence of an elusive but ever-present systemic aspect to local events. Drawing on "the authority of death that lies at the source of the story-form" (Taussig 1997, 77), I bring apparently unrelated or contradictory subject matter (north/south, intimacy/institutions, risk/crime) within one framework, searching for clusters and edges of meaning. The space between stories is unformed. Nevertheless, each space has a moral valence, a capacity to unite, react, or interact with readers' ideas and beliefs. Valences shift as we sense frictions and coincidences in plot, tone, and setting, both within the book and between book and world. Shifting valences lend insights into the vast network of intersecting communicative and biological agents that compose the systemic aspect of global AIDS, its retro political unconscious, its mutant fluidity. This is a species-level event, and we need polyvalent species-level thinking. We need thinking that is capable of accounting for the source and effect of hierarchy and diversity in everyday life; thinking that is open to the unpredictability of trauma, idiosyncratic fury, carnival, and storms at sea; thinking that moves us toward peace.

The Art of a Telling and the Science of Risk

The most telling set of differences occurs between the experts who create categories and schemas for government action and the ordinary people who are affected by them. My aim is to work from what I observed and heard of everyday experience and use this understanding to articulate the issues and perspectives that the experts will not. The AIDS literature is replete with cries about the gap between knowledge and behavior: the question of why individuals continue risking death even after they know about the virus and how it is transmitted (for example, Stall et al. 1990). The expert public health explanation often rests with individual irrationality or incompetence, or the inadequacy of educational strategies. They usually ignore the impact of how bad law and policy can put entire populations at risk. There is, however, growing acknowledgment in the anthropological literature regarding the history of disinformation and distrust between the experts and the people; of the limits of scientific knowledge; and most important, of the existential crises of poverty and violence that overwhelm attempts to reduce risk (for example, Farmer, Connors, and Simmons 1996; Farmer, Lindenbaum, and Good 1993).[10] Less is written about the experts: how their good intentions are skewed by adherence to principles and models that match funding criteria most closely and that are adaptable to the needs of their own careers and bureaucratic organizations. Few talk about how the need for feasibility and accountability may limit the impact of programs, or how loyal adherence to priorities that protect one group or one set of values may imply sacrifice of those who are unrecognized. The point here is not to lay blame, but rather to instigate a change in orientation. We are *all* so caught up in the complex personal and institutional forces that shape our decisions and actions that it is easy for us to lose sight of the biological realities of HIV transmission and infection, or at least to be extremely selective about what we do see. From the viral point of view, the division between expert and layperson may be irrelevant. When, in the book, the statistics of the epidemiologist confront the attitudes of the police and when the injector poses with the square, their elegant scientific solutions, bottom lines, and moral codes may make interesting human drama. But when I insert the perspective of HIV, all the tensions of human difference don't mean a thing, except insofar as they reveal open channels between bloodstreams.

Freed from the sites and methods of collection, I organize the stories according to thematic resonances that come to rest in the three social domains that I refer to as work, escape, and crime. The material comes from three research projects. The first, a big multicity National Institute of Drug Abuse demonstration project, was my introduction to AIDS intervention. In 1988, I was hired on to a team of urban street ethnographers, medical professionals, statisticians, and community outreach workers targeting drug injectors and their sex partners. We had field stations in neighborhoods dominated by the illegal drug and prostitution trades in Chicago. The project got underway well after HIV had a solid grip on the social networks we observed. By 1990, I was in Belize (with side trips to Guatemala) working solo on my second AIDS intervention project. At this time, there had been few reports of people dying of AIDS in Belize, although most people knew about the U.S. epidemic via mass-mediated images and statistics. The atmosphere was thick with rumor. As there are many potential circuits of HIV transmission between Belize and U.S. urban centers like New York and Los Angeles, and between Belize and neighboring countries like Mexico and Honduras, which had begun documenting escalating AIDS rates, it seemed to me to be an auspicious moment to start pulling together some background knowledge for future AIDS prevention efforts, should the Belizean government be prepared to launch them. The third research project did not take place at a geographical field site. Rather, I traveled through cyberspace in search of crime.

The first two parts of the book, "Work" and "Escape," are composed of material intertwined from the Chicago and Belize projects, both of which wed ethnographic methods to a more or less traditional public health framework. Both projects focus on areas of central concern in AIDS prevention—the relationships and risk behaviors of those persons whose lives are dominated, either directly or indirectly, by sex and injected drugs. Chapters 2 and 4, the alpha and omega of "Work," concentrate on prostitution, examining women's use of their bodies as a means of earning money. These chapters contrast the cement ghettos of North America with the tropical periphery of Central America, characterizing the ways in which political and economic inequalities structure the nature and extent of individual risk. The words of Jacqui lead us in.[11] A graceful harbinger of AIDS' future, she demonstrates resilience and intelligence in the face of brutality. Through Jacqui's mind's eye, we glimpse the cold landscape in the shadow of the elevated train tracks where she was servicing her tricks that Chicago autumn. Even as she confirms our worst expectations—her first sexual experience was a violent assault when she was a child and now she turns about thirty-two hundred tricks a year—she serves as a model of professional discipline: she always uses condoms with tricks and does not use hard drugs. This young woman should be busy going to college, I think, but instead she's busy with the cops. At least it's warm in Belize, where the Latina women from surrounding war-torn countries temporarily come to gather down payments for businesses, homes, and college tuition back home, always using condoms with their clients, most of whom are British soldiers, but some tourists and locals, as well; some say Belizean women don't enter the profession, but have sex only with men who are friends or lovers. This is the business of desire, of body parts and fluid collection, mundane physicalities transformed with rituals of charm. And it is the business of our most respected institutions—educational, religious, military—to assure the continuation of these scenes in which tragedy is always a relative thing.

Between these chapters on sex work is a chapter that focuses on work of a different kind, the work of consciousness, of what people have to do to acknowledge the epidemic as a problem. I call it folk surveillance (Chapter 3), the process by which ordinary folks figure out that this virus is relevant to their lives. It is especially important in countries like Belize, where public health institutions might not be doing much in the way of testing blood and documenting cases of HIV disease and death for official surveillance records. Despite all the magical and religious beliefs that exist in the diverse cultures of the Americas, despite our faith in scientific probabilities, there is a strong tendency among many humans to believe this disease is personally relevant only when someone with whom we have a connection gets sick or dies. We do not believe information that's filtered through the media. But if we wait for recognizable symptoms of immune suppression indirectly resulting from HIV disease to appear before us, we wait too long. We've got to believe what science has to say about this invisible beast. Our struggles against racism and colonialism cannot prevent us from making the changes we need to make to stay alive.

The power of ritual to overcome loss is the opening theme of Part 2 of the book, "Escape." Chapter 5, "Death Rites," takes place in Belize. In it, I describe a funeral event, using it as a vehicle to consider what will happen in Belize if prevention fails. How will people come to terms with this new form of death? Even the most traditional ritual forms will have to accommodate the epidemic; this work of accommodation had yet to be accomplished at the time I did fieldwork.

The stress and strain of work, or lack of it, create the need for escape. The next three chapters in Part 2 are basically about getting high and having wildly celebratory casual sex (not necessarily at the same time). Chapters 6 and 7 are about how heroin and cocaine addiction contribute to the level of HIV risk that individuals and communities sustain. Drawing on the life histories of five women in Chicago, these two chapters evoke the mundane side of the drug war, the women's side of war, the after-the-party's-over side. Their life histories are composed of narrative fragments, which are distorted by memory, strategies of self-representation, and joy in the art of telling a good tale. Such distortions raise questions about the blurred line between fact and fiction. The contrast between the women and myself raises questions about the way audience, mission, and credentials shape the authority of ethnographic accounts.

Chapter 8, "Easter in Livingston," is about a Good Friday procession, partying for days and nights on end on a Caribbean beach in the heart of what feels like Africa—an unusual tourist destination on the coast of Guatemala. The events provoke thinking on the varieties of sexual behavior, the transnationality of sex, and the incalculability of HIV risk when the public spirit enters the carnivalesque. So ends our "Escape."

By this time readers should realize that for most of us there is no escape. It's enough to make you turn to Part 3 of the book, "Crime." Despite north-south maneuvers, the first two parts of the book present the pandemic in classic ethnographic terms, that is, knowledge gained through dialogue and participant observation in specific cultural locales with a focus on prevention. In the third part, I forfeit the sense of being in a local culture in order to pull data from more diffuse channels. I take in appellate court transcripts as a member of a dispersed and faceless cohort of researchers and chroniclers, and television and newspaper stories as a lone member of a mass audience. Like John Fiske (1994), I keep an eye out for media events that give form and presence to an already existing discursive current out there in the world—the criminalization of intentional HIV transmission. And following Jameson (1994, 347), I imagine the media as a collective actor on the historical scene.

By presenting this topic for popular consumption and legal debate, the media oversee a phantasmagoric transformation of HIV from parasite to weapon. The modulation of HIV as an imaginative figure involves a shift in the focus of attention. As the primary subjects of AIDS intervention in the public health mode, the uninfected move into the background. In step the subjects of legal intervention, the already HIV-infected. More particularly, the focus is on HIV-positive persons who are said to have knowingly and willingly infected others.

This is a taboo subject among many AIDS activists, although it has been raised as a warning that homophobic forces of evil and ignorance continue to gather strength (for example, Watney 1994), or less directly, as a psychosocial problem of self-disclosure (for example, Sobo 1995). Most legal scholars whom I have read more or less agree that criminalization is unfair and unethical, and not only will it not work to stop HIV transmission, but it will most likely damage the public trust so necessary for voluntary testing, the touchstone of surveillance and early treatment.[12]

I do not disagree. Nevertheless, I persist in a cultural analysis of the subject for two reasons. The first is that I don't think the push for criminalization will disappear just because scholars and activists wish it away. Although in 1996, public comment succeeded in convincing the U.S. Sentencing Commission that a federal law criminalizing HIV transmission remains unwise, this victory pales before the proliferation of new HIV-specific laws at the state level: Between 1986 and 1996 there were eighty HIV-specific laws passed either in state houses and / or senates, the majority of which make specific reference to sexual behavior.[13]

Second, I think that the subject of intentional HIV transmission reveals much about the political unconscious of AIDS that cannot be traced to homophobia alone. Moral conundrums raised by questions of crime may lend insight into the ways in which citizens in democratic states seek out the force of law to control fearful aspects of social change. They also offer insight into the ways in which the media propel stories into the in boxes on state prosecutors' desks and help inspire the passage of new legislation and more intensive police power. The connection between law and social change has to be examined in the context of ordinary social life (Falk Moore 1973, 78). For better or worse, mass media's information and exaggerations are an influential part of the process.

I do not trace the lines of legal argument at issue here, but rather, I present a range of human experiences that together characterize the phenomena. This is by no means a comprehensive account, as there are certain categories of HIV-related crime that are not included (for example, rape, sex with minors, needle stickups, biting and spitting in penal settings). I select stories that for the most part involve sexually related passions gleaned from field notes, media accounts, and courtroom transcripts, passions that struggle for and against the state, or passions that play out against the background of a state-in-waiting (the entertainment state, the state prison).

I approach the topic with trepidation, as it's easier to talk about people whom I can believe are basically good than to grapple with the shocking unpleasantries of intentional evil, or our strange desire to fantasize about it. HIV has entered the political unconscious, where it assumes the guise of a biological weapon and inspires new forms of crime. While this topic is peopled with all types, Chapters 9 through 12 focus primarily on persons engaged in unsafe, consensual sex, where one person hides his or her HIV-positive status from the other. Conspiracy, psychopathology, abuse, and alienation are the usual accompaniments to these kinds of events. Together, criminal cases and the many new laws that impel their prosecution may also be framed as a kind of AIDS prevention, one that operates as a backup to prevention in the public health mode.

Chapter 9, "Desperate," addresses the thorny issue of cases in which malice may overshadow necessity among some HIV-positive prostitutes who continue working. The coding of deviant bodies and sexual subjects in the law has a long history of unequal application that makes the handling of this issue complex and contradictory, as does the merging of what we usually think of as victim and perpetrator within the same body. The topic is an apt one for demonstrating Carol Smart's (1995) argument that law is a gendering strategy. In contrast, some people are above the law. Chapter 10, "The Positively Arrogant Mishap," is about how AIDS secrecy nearly destroyed an economically successful American Buddhist community. Like Chapters 3 and 5 on folk surveillance and death rites, the narrative of these events grapples with the subject of how traditional beliefs must grow to accommodate changing biological realities, even when such change contradicts the most fundamental aspects of belief. As these events show, resistance to change can be fatal. Chapter 11, "Outtakes," is about the wild extremes of human imagination and action—needle attacks, the woman scorned meets the brotherhood of the doomed, mass suicide. Chapter 12, "Everything I Have Is Yours," the title borrowed from a popular jazz tune, is about heterosexuals who may purposely try to infect their partners. This topic lends itself to analysis of fictional and documentary television genres and their dynamic relationship with the anxious norm, a region of human emotion located at the paradoxical intersection of pleasure and fear, a market niche for mass entertainment. People who fit the anxious norm might worry that intimates may in fact be strangers who take advantage of vulnerability and naiveté. Instead of having open conversations about their concerns with their partners, people who fit the anxious norm might instead seek fictions to displace their fears on evil characters who can be contained by the state, thereby feeding their personal panic as well as the public impulse for punitiveness.

While the section on crime focuses on the bad acts of a few individuals, the impact of their deeds (and the impact that the interventions of criminal law might have on the interventions of public health more generally) must be weighed against potential damage caused by institutional practices. As Hannah Arendt (1964) reminds us, it is not intentional acts of evil but unintentional acts socialized by institutions that must be combated. Governmental institutions responsible for health, education, and justice must change the way they function since they either contribute directly to the spread of HIV (as does the U.S. justice system) or contribute indirectly by accommodating drug war priorities. If institutions change the conditions under which *populations* engage in HIV risk behaviors, the fatal consequences of *individual* choice in global HIV transmission patterns will diminish markedly.

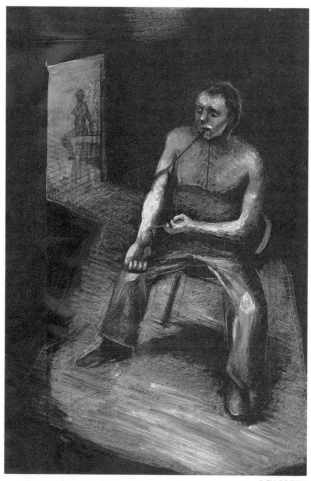

PART I   *Work*

Passion and
panicked blurs
of colors and
sleepless dreams.
Lying naked
in a moss marsh
as water color
etchings form in sand.

Death's not
like a soaring
owl but rumbles
like trembling
limbs, quaking
loins.
A little like a
lover's sigh
a friend's laughter.

—*C. Jason Dotson*

2 / Prostitution North

By the time the federal government's street-based AIDS research and intervention project targeting Chicago's drug injectors was well established, nearly one out of four whose blood was tested was positive for HIV antibodies.[1] A growing concern for those whom injectors might be infecting through sex led to my being hired as an ethnographer focusing on their sex partners, which was a new epidemiological risk category. The multicity project was the scientific outgrowth of the late 1980s panic that the epidemic might spread from stigmatized risk groups to the so-called general population. Conceived in Washington, D.C., as the female non-injecting counterpart of male injectors, the sex partners included prostitutes who did not shoot drugs. Project field sites were chosen precisely because they were central copping areas for (male) injectors, so we found few prostitutes who did not shoot drugs. Field stations were set up at each site, and recovering addicts were hired as outreach workers. They created and nurtured the crucial communication channels ethnographers depended upon to find people willing to talk about illegal behaviors (Sterk-Elifson 1993).

Forty-seventh Street and Martin Luther King Drive is a busy intersection in the heart of Chicago's southside. It is also the location of the field station administered and staffed by African Americans to target the African American community. (Just as Latinos were hired

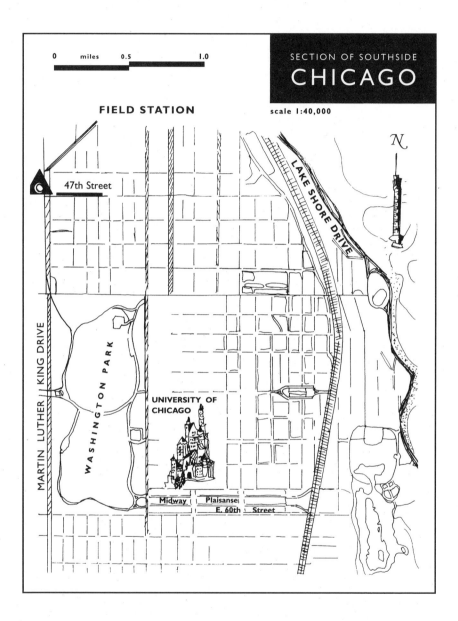

SECTION OF SOUTHSIDE
CHICAGO

FIELD STATION   scale 1:40,000

0   miles   0.5   1.0

47th Street

LAKE SHORE DRIVE

N

MARTIN LUTHER KING DRIVE

WASHINGTON PARK

UNIVERSITY OF CHICAGO

Midway   Plaisanse
E. 60th   Street

to reach the Mexican and Puerto Rican communities on the westside and whites were hired to reach the predominantly white communities on the northside.) Fifty years ago, the neighborhood around the southside field station was a booming center of diverse economic activity (Drake and Clayton 1970). By 1990, over half the people in the area were below the poverty line. The cement towers of Robert Taylor Homes are nearby. One of the largest housing projects in the United States, it is home to tens of thousands of people who can barely glimpse the economic horizons enjoyed by those in the glass and steel towers in the center city loop (Johnson 1994). The illicit drug and sex trade has devoured this landscape and many of its people, and HIV is raging.

George Lewis, also known as Loki, was an outreach worker for the project. He has since died. Loki's memory evokes in me the intense mixture of joy and pain, artfulness and decadence, that characterized my experience of being with folks in and around the southside field station. He was a talented toast-teller.[2] Although we didn't work together regularly, he did line up Jacqui, my first interview. Excerpts from field notes and interview transcripts offer a sense of the narratives of hardship I recorded.[3]

They knocked on his door at two in the morning asking for condoms. The twenty-two-year-old woman and her man worked across the street from Loki's house in the south Sixties of Chicago. Angry about being awakened, he told them he never has condoms after ten at night. After they left, his conscience got to bothering him, and he got dressed and went downstairs to give them the condoms. The couple had already returned from buying three for two dollars at the drugstore. They were upset about a woman working out there who was HIV-positive and wasn't using any.

Not long after that, Loki brought them into the field station on Forty-Seventh and Martin Luther King Drive. The man stayed in the reception area with their two-month-old baby and the woman came into one of the back rooms to be interviewed. She was a slip of a woman with a gentle, beautiful, bruised face, and the raggediest skirt and blouse I'd ever seen outside of the bus terminal in Peshawar. She said that she didn't inject drugs and her man didn't either. But half her tricks did and she did about ten tricks a night. Without counting for time off and seasonal variation, that was a total of about thirty-two hundred tricks a year.

First we went through the government's quantitative surveillance interview. I learned that she was a bisexual, Baptist, high school grad. She worked sex full-time and had her own apartment, which she shared with her man and her two-month-old child. She also had a two-year-old who didn't live with them. Her drug use history was limited to occasional alcohol and marijuana. The majority of her clients were men, although she also performed unprotected oral sex on women. She knew that at least nine men and six women clients were injectors. Like most of the prostitutes I talked to, she reported using condoms with everyone except her boyfriend. She began this discipline three months after she started sex work as a result of a case of gonorrhea. She was in good health; she found herself in jail about once a week; she had donated or sold blood after 1979. With this interview completed, we tape recorded a free-form life history interview focusing on sex and drug-related HIV risk. I asked her what it was like the first time she had sex, a standard opener. I was unprepared for what she said [my questions and interjections are in brackets]:

■ When I first had sex I was raped. [By whom?] I don't know. [Some guy on the street?] I was coming home from the store. He asked me, he said, "Have you seen a ring, a diamond ring around here on the ground?" I said, "No." So he said, "Well, can you help me look for it?" I was ten years old, I said, "Okay, I'll help you look for it." He said, "If you find it for me I'll give you seven dollars." I said, "Okay." So the seven dollars perked up my urge for helping this man find this ring. So he said, "Well come on over and walk over here to this store with me." So I walked over to the store. The store happened to be by an alley. So we got in front of the store, he grabbed me and pulled me in back of the alley and told me to be quiet. It was some little kids back there and I hollered. So he twisted my ear and he gagged my mouth and he started choking me and took me down to the basement. He raped me and all, blood started coming out of me. He raped me front and back. That was the first time. Then after then I just been wide opened. [What do you mean?] My vagina haven't closed back from that cause I was ripped and he was real big, he was a real big guy. . . .

They took me to the hospital and they tried to look for the guy. Right now today I see this same guy around my parents' house. The first time I seen him again, my father ran over there and beat him with a bat. They called the police and they had him locked up and a few hours later he was out walking the streets again. Ever since then, I been having sex. I started working on the street about a year and a half ago. I met this guy, the one that is here with me now, he was telling me how it was and it all sounded so good coming from the mouth. You get out on the street and it's a different thing.

Jacqui liked the guy she was with, and he asked her to catch tricks for him so she said okay. She isn't looking for another kind of work, because this money is faster than any of the straight jobs available to her. At $15 to $20 for a five- to six-minute job with condom only, she clears an average of $150 to $200 a night off-the-books. The condoms are negotiated up front, along with price and sex act. When I asked if her clients give her flack, she recounted this event. It took place in a drunk's car near the stroll on Seventieth and Western:

■ Yes. . . . Sometimes they will say, okay [they'll use a condom], and then when we start to date, they will try and slip it off. And when they slip it off, I leave. I take the money and everything and leave. I still have static with them and so we get on the street and we get to arguing and stuff like that. Just like a man bit me in my face right there. . . . He bit me, about forty dollars, a white guy. . . . He wanted a half and half, right. [What does that mean?] That consists of oral and regular sex. [But he only comes once? He starts in the mouth and he switches, or the other way around?] Right. He said he was suppose to get two satisfaction, two nut full [orgasms], right. So I said, "Nah." So he said, "Well bitch give me my money back!" I said, "Nah it's not happening like that." I tried to grab the door and get out . . . he grabs me right here in my face with his teeth and just start biting. It hurt and I bit him back. So we both got marks.

[So do you have all kinds of people coming to you, like white guys, black guys, Hispanic guys?] Yes. [You have regular customers?] I stopped having regular customers, because regular customers are more problems than just picking a guy off the street. Because a regular customer, he tends to want deals, he wants to give you half the money this time. Half the money next time. Some of them will fall in love with you. I had a couple of them that fell in love with me. I had to leave them alone. They would come down while I'm working and acting crazy and what not. Telling me to get off the street and pulling me, pulling my clothes and what not. I had a lot of them like that before. This life is crazy, believe it or not.

Whether on southside, westside, or northside strolls, Jacqui said that tricks come by all night long—although the south Sixties area tends to have more women than tricks. If she doesn't run out of money in the daytime, she'll start work about eleven at night and stay out until five in the morning. Tricks be out there all night, she said. Most come out after two in the morning and stay out till seven. They be out there, these men with jobs and wives:

■   . . . especially on the weekends. I just see more traffic at night on weekends than you do in the daytime, because everybody be at work during the daytime and they come out during weekends to go party. When they come from their party, they are ready to go out and have sex with somebody. Be different sex instead of going home to their wife. Some of them may just want to come out and just get a blow job or something. I used to have this one guy, this young guy in the winter-time, every day, he's about seventeen years old. Every day he give me twenty dollars just to lick my toes and that felt good in the wintertime, my feet would be so cold.

Outside Castle University[4]

I didn't see the stroll across from Loki's house until the end of October. We were in his car. Jacqui was out there working alongside another woman. Loki asked Jacqui's man about the other woman's pimp. As Loki was approaching the wrong man, the woman's pimp pulled up in a car. Loki got out to talk to him. The pimp wore a leather cap painted gold, he was big and really stoned, eyes bleary, voice slack and definitely not to mess with. It was cold. Loki invited them into his car. We were in the front and they got in the back. Loki explained the project. Hoping for a warm break, the woman asked if they could go to the station for an interview. Loki said he didn't make no arrangements with the woman; it was the man he talked to. Loki addressed the man, eventually getting him to agree to come. They followed us in their car as we tried to drop Loki's son off at the baby-sitter a couple of blocks away. She wasn't there, so they followed us back to his house. I stayed in the car while Loki took his son inside and called the field station to make sure we could bring them. We couldn't because it was time for the field station staff meeting. So the pimp and the pro left. We hoped that they would come around again next Friday, but they didn't show.

Waiting in the car I got a good look at the stroll. It ran dark and cold under the El. Between the El and the end of the row of houses that included Loki's, there were empty lots of broken glass and dried

WORK

city weeds. Abandoned storefronts of a once lively neighborhood held heaped up garbage, and here and there, a mattress for working women to use.

Cold, dirty, broken glass, and no water—these are the conditions under which the women who work this southside stroll endure. Just a very few blocks north of here, a five- to ten-minute walk, is that wide and regal greensward, lined with the stone spires of Rockefeller money, the campus of the University of Chicago. What keeps this rich city of knowledge so immune from the desperate poverty surrounding? Certainly police patrols help. But how is it that some of the richness doesn't flow over to the surround, an adventurous restaurant here, a new laundromat there? The differences of privilege and poverty entrenched in this landscape have worked their ways into the very bloodstreams of its inhabitants. Here I was working with someone from the neighborhood to try to intervene in a situation that seemed overdetermined by a long history of inequality. Paid by the National Institute of Drug Abuse through the auspices of the University of Illinois, there seemed to be no clear path through the treacherous morass of government-sponsored do-gooding.

Institutional Change

I never did get used to these interviews. I have two reasons for presenting parts of Jacqui's personal history here. The first is to convey a sense of the street world from a young sex worker's perspective. This function has been central to the proliferation of ethnographic accounts that have accompanied AIDS research and intervention projects. Accounts of experience fill in the empty categories that are the basic tools of epidemiologists. They provide data for analysis of broader social processes. They provide ballast for statistics whose numerical significance may be independent of human significance. In a more general sense, they nudge reform forward.

My second reason for presenting her story is a more ambivalent one. Together, quantitative and ethnographic descriptions of groups at risk for HIV create a domain of meaning that becomes the dominant reference point for intervention. The creators and arbiters of this domain are well funded to simulate a source of truth and accountability for professionals dealing with epidemic management. As new risk groups are added to the semantic domain of investigation, it's continually replenished. As it became clear that it wasn't just gays, injectors, hemophiliacs, and their sex partners who were at risk, instead of abandoning the fiction of an immune general public safely cordoned off from the marked risk groups in their midst, epidemic managers just kept adding new groups to target: women, minorities, fetuses, adolescents, rural and suburban residents (Glick-Schiller 1992). The new target groups tend to be those sectors of society that are amenable to operationalization by researchers, and they tend to leave out other possible groups that are harder to identify, such as bisexuals, gay black men, and generic married couples. The epidemiological model is always full enough to convey the reassuring illusion that the government has things under control. In fact, however, alongside the universe of quantitative and qualitative descriptions of people at risk is a universe of unasked questions.

AIDS research and intervention is a form of surveillance, even when (or especially when) it is carried out with the benefit of the target population in mind. Those in power do the watching, the others are watched. The aim of public health is cramped within the limits of public acceptability and commitment in an antidrug-crazed era. The only thing our intervention project could do for Jacqui was send her back out on the street with a bunch of free condoms in her pocket. Why were we not mounting an honest and courageous public health intervention that would initiate debates at top government levels on the crucial question of access to clean needles? We document that Jacqui's risk is derived primarily from tricks who inject drugs in a city where carrying a clean needle may make one subject to arrest. She is not unique. By 1996, the Centers for Disease Control and

Prevention (CDC 1997, 565), reported that over one-third (36 percent) of the 573,000 U.S. AIDS cases among adults were directly or indirectly associated with injecting drug use. Why are researchers and educators not making serious efforts to confront misguided or half-hearted needle policies? How have we come to accept the neutralization of our efforts?[5]

The real test of conviction in our struggle to control AIDS is a willingness for government institutions to turn the research gaze upon themselves. To study—not the individuals trapped in the violent and unhealthy conditions that are forced upon poor inner-city dwellers—but to study how the institutions themselves can change, or at least to understand why they won't. In lieu of continuing the costly and pointless routine of forcing sex workers through endless rounds of arrest, court, street, and back again; of chasing them from neighborhood to neighborhood; why not urge police to work at enforcing rape laws? In lieu of using workers' condoms as evidence of a crime, why not urge police to work at protecting women from violent assault?

The constant threat of violence in their personal and professional lives may severely undermine women's determination to reduce HIV-related risk. That Jacqui was raped as a child and bitten as a woman at work may seem like random bad luck at the individual level. But this is just one example of the brutal fact that African Americans, inner-city dwellers, and low-income women in the United States do not have the legal protection from violence that majority citizens take for granted (see Connors 1996 and Gordon 1990, 151–65). The police do a better job of enforcing the structure of violence than in keeping the peace in minority communities like the southside. The threat of AIDS pales in comparison to the risks children take walking to elementary school!

In her critique of the U.S. justice system, Diana Gordon (1990, ix, 10, 242) shows how street crime has become a social problem whose unsolvability created opportunities for academics and practitioners to get challenging and sometimes well-paid work. These professionals pay lip service to the idea that social and economic inequalities are key sources of high rates of assault, yet their solutions rely almost exclusively on a capture and confinement model that discriminates against the poor. By displacing attention to the problem of assessing individual guilt, the public has become less committed to working for larger social policies that can begin to close divisions. We will only change, she says, when we abandon the emphasis on individual guilt as the analytic perspective for understanding crime. The same could be said for understanding health crises such as AIDS. The same nexus of problems that cause crime contribute to the high HIV seroprevalence rates in inner-city communities. Until public health institutions acknowledge their complicity in reproducing social and economic inequality, AIDS prevention efforts will at best remain well-intentioned alibis. We cannot ignore the damage wrought by the institutions dedicated to "justice."

If Jacqui ever entertained the possibility that she might grow up to be a professor down the street at the University of Chicago, she wouldn't be out there "at risk," making "choices" about whether to use condoms or not. Taking AIDS seriously means changing institutional structures of oppression; it means realizing that everyone who is an agent of those structures benefits from them; it means questioning the existence of that unholy divide between Rockefeller's greensward and Jacqui's stroll; it means releasing sexual service from the stigma of criminality. Without institutional change, the virus wins. And that's why most of the money allocated to this epidemic gets poured into the search for a pharmaceutical cure, the magic that will solve the problem while allowing the distribution of power and health to remain more or less the same.

The National Commission on AIDS (1992, 11) has warned: "We cannot continue to teach individuals about the dangers of certain behaviors as if they choose to engage in them indiscriminately. We would do well to take account of social forces and institutions that undermine individuals' capacity to adopt and sustain a healthy life-style. It is difficult to change practices effectively without changing circumstances."

The Fall

Working on the Chicago AIDS project was rough. My job was to carry out ethnography on an epidemiological category that had no social reality. People just didn't acknowledge having sex with a drug injec-tor as a social identity in ordinary circumstances. And in contrast to the research model that conceptualized sex partners as female, half of the sex partners whom we did find turned out to be men. But the structure of these projects was preformed in Washington, D.C., and Washington wanted data on their own terms, not critical feedback demonstrating the weaknesses of nationwide protocols.[6]

To cheer me up, Loki would occasionally tell me a toast or two. On June 27, 1989, my last night in town, he let me record a whole string of toasts from his repertoire. He learned most of them in prison as a young man several decades before I met him. "The Fall" is one toast that captures the spirit of panache crucial to surviving life before the time of AIDS:[7]

> Now some of you guys might be surprised
> of what I'm about to say.
> And you'll say whose that lame who
> says he knows the game
> Now where did he learn to play?
>
> I'd like to tell you a story
> the trick fate played on me.
> If you gather round
> I'm gonna run it down,
> And I'm gonna unravel my history.

It was a Saturday night
and the jungle was bright
as the gamers stalked their prey.
The code was crime
and the neon line
and the weak was doomed to pay.

This is where crime begun
where daughter fought son
and your father stays in jail
and your ma lays woke
with a heart most broke
while the train loads up for hell.

Where addicts prowl
with a tiger's snarl
seeking that lethal blow
and wineheads cringe
on the canned heat binge
and find their graves in the snow.

Where belles of vice
sell love for a price
and even the law is corrupt.
But you keep on tryin'
and you keep on cryin'
sayin' man it's a bitter cup.

Now she was a brown-skinned moll
like a Chinese doll
walkin' the ways of sin
up and down she would trod
with a wink and a nod
to the nearest whorehouse din.

So it wasn't by chance
that I caught her glance
I intended to steal this dame
and I thought with glee
Holy Jesus, it's time for me to gain.

When I hit on the broad
from her eye a teardrop fell
when I asked her why
she began to cry
and told a sad and bitter tale.

All about some guy
who blacks her eyes
take all the money she gets
how she lays in jail
and he won't go her bail
and he dares her to call it quits.

I say, well Baby, dry your tears
and have no fears
for the Kind Lover's here
and I'm staking my claim
in this piece of the game
and I'll vow I'll have no fears.

She looked at me
like a slave set free
and said, "Daddy, I'm your girl."
Her man didn't stir
as I split with her
and we made it all over this world.

She caught on fast
as the months rolled past
and I played her till the bitter end.
A better hoe
I've yet to know
true, they say a dog is a man's best friend.

She ranked with the best
from the east to the west
when her boostin' hand was down,
she stole the knocks out of knees
even Fido's fleas
she thieved out of many a town.

She was a good shot broad
a pro at fraud
The Drag she played like a bet
played stuff like an ace
never lost a case
and put many a chump in debt.

She tricked with Frenchmen,
torpedoes, and hitmen,
to her they were all the same.
She tricked with Jews, Apaches, and Sioux,
and some breeds I can't even name.

She tricked with Greeks, Arabs, freaks,
she tricked in the house of God
and there was no son of a gun
that this one would shun
that could pay and claim a rod.

W O R K

With a lick or a laugh
from her yellow cap
the tricks would fight a duel
my longest bread
was made with her head
and she could really chew.

And she had good round eye
and that's no lie
the whorehouse knew it would swing
And many a nut was bust in her butt
because the rag didn't mean a thing.

Anywhere she would folla
that righteous dolla
to hell if she had to go
and be down their waitin'
to trick with ole Satan
my God, she was already gettin' low.

Now I've heard whores cry
about the wind being high
and the man being on their tail,
about snow and sleet being asshole deep
and the tricks can go to hell.

And a greasy spoon
or a jukebox saloon
you find 'em killing time.
Cryin' hard luck tales
and suckin' up bails
the pimps ain't gettin' a dime.

Yardin', slidin', Rayfieldin', hidin',
suckin' them party pricks
and noddin' so tough
for fuckin' with stuff
she can't see no mother-fuckin' tricks.

You can cop her lid
for the lowest bid
you can set her ass on fire.
You can dig in her cunt
for a mother-fuckin' month
she's the cheapest bitch you can hire.

And the rents been due for a month or two
and the landlord's hoppin' mad.
The bitch would ease between your sheets
with no night receipts and tell you
"Daddy, the night was bad."

And on Monday for sure
you can find that whore
'cause some lame beat walker caught her.
And you pawn your shit
to get her ripped
while the bitch ain't made a quarter.

But you pay a price
when you deal in vice
we all know it takes a steady grind
and a whore had to get up and go
to beat this triple-a bitch of mine.

W O R K

Like a sex machine
she walked between raindrops snow and hail
standin' on hot bricks
she lured them tricks
come blizzard, cyclone, and gale.

Now the trouble began
when I stopped smokin' and started to hit.
cause you know I blew more dope
than any one whore could git.

I blowed my shack
my Cadillac
the rugs right off my floor
I pawned my ice
for a hell of a price
and shot up all that dope.

I stole from Ma, swung Pa,
and sold my pedigree pup
pawned my treads
sold my bed
and shot the TV up.

My woman cried
and damn near died
when I made off with her mink
but I stayed in my role
and stole' and sold
everything but the kitchen sink.

Now, the real trouble begins
when the girl took sick
and couldn't gin

she had the piles
the inflamed biles
for a month she couldn't pee.
When her ovaries failed
I was shocked to hell
cause things really looked bad for me.

When lockjaw set in,
believe me, friend,
the Chinaman took his toll.
Her head was dead,
her ass was red,
and the lips on her cunt was cold.

So down I fell
to the depths of hell
I put myself in the cross.
My habit stood tall
and my money got small
and everything I had was lost.

But I wanted to be fair
and on the square
I didn't want to ditch the broad.
So I said, what the hell,
the bitch ain't well
I'll get her a wife-in-law.

I said, "Baby, you lay right there
till you're feelin' fine
and you can get back on the street.
And I'm gonna do my best
while you convalesce
and can get you back on your feet.

There's a little young bitch
with a whorehouse itch
that I could probably latch on to
and there's that redhead whore
that's ready to go,
if the deal's O.K. with you."

Now there's not a whore in the game
whose got the name
for kickin' the mud you kick.
So you lay right there
till you're feelin' fair
then we gonna climb on out of this clip.

You take a broad like this
was a good man's bitch
she had everything it took.
There's just one thought
once she's caught
the bitch won't loose the hook.

Hell no! she said.
I'll see you dead
before I'll let you go.
And the black coach of sorrow
'll pick your ass up tomorrow
if you walk beyond that door.

I lost my health
in a bid for wealth
so you could play your bit.
But you went dope head
and blowed the bread
now you talkin' that stable shit.

I'm hip to the way all you pimps
play on the loves you drop on the trail.
But I'm gonna call the police
if this bullshit don't cease
and bury your slick ass in jail.

(Ha!)
Now I laughed at this dame
and her jilted claim
while leapin' from the bed
while packin' my shit
and fixin' to split
this is what I said:

Bitch, you ain't no lame
you know the game,
they call it cop and blow.
You've had your run
now you're done
I'm gonna get me another hoe.

I can't make no swag
on no swayback nag
and your thoroughbred days are past.
Well wouldn't I look silly
puttin' a cripple filly
on a track that's much too fast.

So get out of my way
I'm fixin' to split
I mean get the fuck off my back,
cause I'll need some dough
and I've got to have a hoe
that you run on a speedy track.

Now while layin' all back
in another broad's shack
about to cop a plea
I heard a thunder
that the door shook under
wonder what the fuck can that be?

In stepped the nailer
on his face was a grin
mixed with a deadly expression
he said if your name is Loki
Pimpin' Loki
all you've got to do is sign this confession.

And the bitch stood there
with her finger in the air
That's him! That's him!
she cried with glee.
That's the son of a bitch
with a con man's pitch
that made a whore out of me.

A crashin' blow
sent me to the floor
I was sunk in a backward pose.
When I woke
my jaw was broke
and blood was all over my clothes.

That just goes to show
that the strongest hoe
can give in to that female simpin'

and a bitch wasn't born
without the female scorn
I was booked on two counts of pimpin'.

In a six-by-six cell
in the Cook County Jail
I watched the sun rise in the East
and the morning stills
and the jungle chills
give sleep to the slumbering beast.

Farewell to the nights
and the neon lights
farewell I say to it all.
Farewell to the game
may it still be the same
next year when I'm through doing this fall.

3 / Folk Surveillance

If you don't know anyone who has died of it, believing that AIDS can kill you is like believing in ghosts. That's what it seemed like in 1990 Belize. Occasionally spliced between *700 Club* Christian vaudeville-news shows and old *Hazel* reruns, televised images of gaunt-faced North Americans suffering with AIDS beamed into living rooms up and down the Caribbean coast. A few local people had experienced the confusing array of AIDS-related symptoms, but they did not fit the persistent and inaccurate stereotype linking HIV exclusively to gay white men. In this time and place, AIDS had yet to become a social fact. Perhaps, by some miracle, it never would.

The Cultural Locale

Belize is an ethnically and linguistically diverse nation that borders a long string of coral reef on the Central American coast of the Caribbean Sea (part of the same formation upon which the sailboat *Meriah* met her end). British Honduras, once a superior refuge for pirates and a source of tropical hardwoods, gained its independence and became Belize in 1981. Blacks are in the majority, dominating the upper echelons of business and government while also filling the poorest ranks. Most blacks are English-speaking Creoles, an ethnic identification that blurs black-white racial distinctions. A minority are Garifuna, descendants of Africans and Arawak Indians who speak their own language as well as English. Living peacefully with the Creoles and Garifuna are the Kekchi, Mopan, and Yucatec Mayan Indians, each with their own language. There are also East Indians whose ancestors were brought from India by the British to work in the fields; a population of Chinese that had been growing rapidly when I was there, with the families of businessmen and women leaving Hong Kong. There are so many Spanish-speaking immigrants from the surrounding nations of Guatemala, Mexico, Honduras, and El Salvador, that some Belizeans had begun to worry about the weakening hold of English as the national language. There are still a lot of British of one sort or another who continue to profit from their investments, and plenty of folks from the United States, whose dollar has become the official national currency. There are almost as many religions as there are ethnic identities. People relate in many different ways to the Catholic Church, which is not only the dominant religious institution, but a moral and economic force influencing secular institutions such as education and health. Ethnic, linguistic, and religious diversity combine to make Belizean identity rich and dynamic. As many folks pointed out to me, sexual culture operates in the mix. There is too much interethnic dating going on to use ethnicity as a marker for tracing HIV transmission risk.

Tourism and agriculture are the two major engines of development, the former capitalizing on Belize's beautiful ocean and forest treasures, the latter on the sun, land, fresh water, and cheap labor. Both industries are susceptible to epidemiological analysis: tourism because it brings in sexually active persons from epidemic epicenters such as New York and Los Angeles and because it actively promotes sexual interaction as a central element in the tropical paradise vacation; agriculture because it depends directly on male migrant laborers and indirectly on female prostitutes, most of whom, I suspect, do not receive health and education benefits conducive to HIV risk reduction.

Belize City, located where the dirty mouth of the Belize River

47

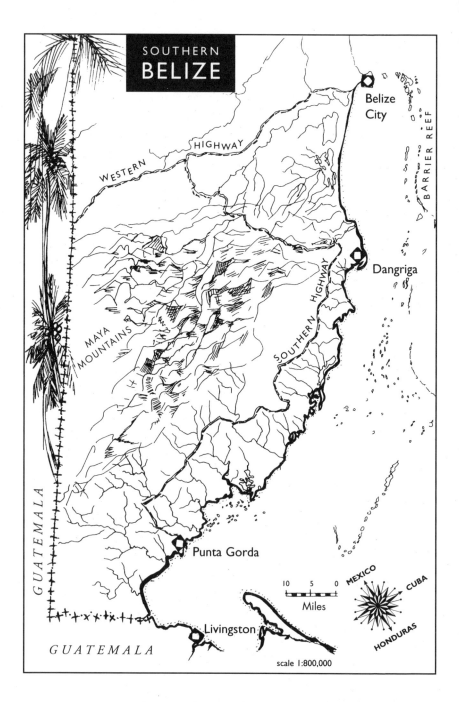

SOUTHERN
BELIZE

Belize
City

BARRIER REEF

WESTERN HIGHWAY

SOUTHERN HIGHWAY

Dangriga

MAYA
MOUNTAINS

GUATEMALA

Punta Gorda

10   5   0

Miles

MEXICO   CUBA

HONDURAS

Livingston

GUATEMALA

scale 1:800,000

empties into the sea, is the biggest city in this nation of about two hundred thousand people. 1990 was the year of the city's first elevator. But neither the modern conveniences offered by an optimistic tourist industry nor the well-kept white balustrades reminiscent of British empire hid the poverty from anyone who cared to look. Just about all the homes in the city had water and electricity, but walk a couple of miles in any direction away from a hotel and you would find a neighborhood that hauled away its sewage in plastic buckets. Many were dumped directly in the open waterways lining the streets. Scrubbing their houses spotless and covering their flower-printed furniture in plastic, homemakers were dismayed by ever-present flies.

When I wasn't in Belize City, most of my time was spent in Punta Gorda, a small town of about two thousand souls representing a cross-section of ethnic groups, with Garifuna and Maya (many of whom live in surrounding villages) forming the area's majorities. Punta Gorda, or "PG" as it is called, is strategically located near the southern coastal border with Guatemala. This has resulted in the dubious distinction of being home to an intercontinental Voice of America station. Just south of town, this impressive array of steel spires sheds surreal light against the night jungle and sea surround, its acoustic signals coding foreign patriotism unheard by passersby. To the north is the not uncommon noise of exploding hills, soldiers fanning out from the British army base just west of town to fire their weapons in the rain as they wait for a hypothetical Guatemalan invasion.

Official and Semiofficial AIDS Surveillance

The disjunctures of late-twentieth-century images, products, and diseases passing through this old hideout of pirates, Indians, freed slaves, petite bourgeois, and independent spirits is startling. Still, AIDS prevention posters could not bear the image of a condom. Still, the Red Cross respected the beliefs of the Catholic Church and

49

taught only abstinence in its school AIDS prevention programs. Still, the World Health Organization's man in Belize kept reporting only eleven or twelve AIDS cases a year.[1]

Of course, Nurse Woods of the Belize City Sexually Transmitted Disease (STD) clinic knew better. She had been trying to keep track, but she'd gone to Jamaica for a year, with the cumulative stats in her head. Nurse Peters, her replacement, went through the recent records for me when I interviewed her on February 7.

The previous November was a bad month. There were two HIV-positive cases the first week, both from Honduras: a twenty-year-old woman with a seronegative child and a man who said he had contact with a female prostitute in a Guatemala-Belize border town. Later that month, two people with AIDS died two days apart. The previous week a baby and a man suspected of having AIDS died. The clinic routinely gave HIV antibody tests to every client. The hospitals were also supposed to report their cases to Nurse Peters so that she could keep track of national stats, but they didn't. Like the deaths she'd heard about last week, she'd had no time to track them down. According to the records she had, it looked like 19 dead. Of the 477 tested as part of the regular STD clinic in the previous seventeen weeks, 9 (1.9 percent), were positive. This sample was drawn principally from native Belizeans. In contrast, of the 68 people who sought testing to fulfill Belizean immigration requirements, 22.5 percent tested HIV-positive. This rate almost matches the southside Chicago sample of drug injectors tested in 1988!

The over tenfold difference in AIDS case numbers that the STD clinic sample found between Belizean native and immigrant groups is reflected in the regional surveillance stats published by WHO for that year. The 1990–1991 stats list Belize's 12 AIDS cases (an intentional underestimate) along with 8,720 from Mexico; 1,306 from Honduras; 370 from El Salvador; and 176 from Guatemala (WHO 1991).[2] The estimated number of people infected with HIV but not showing symptoms is, of course, many times higher. Regional differences may be due to a number of factors, including variations in the extent and kind of AIDS surveillance, accuracy of census data, and honesty of reporting. Nevertheless, the comparison provides some insight into the more general patterns about which Nurses Peters and Woods were concerned. Clearly, the fiction that national borders can contain AIDS cannot be sustained for long.

Future Shock

What sticks to you longer than a girlfriend?
—*Belizean* AIDS *joke*

I spoke to many people about AIDS as I traveled up and down the coast between Belize City and PG. I was trying to get a sense of how people ordered their perceptions of the global pandemic that was for the most part still swirling outside their nation's porous borders. Fragments of conversations reconstructed from field notes about the initial set of AIDS cases to hit public consciousness contain the makings of a folk surveillance. The words convey a watchfulness that blurs science and suspicion, pathology and cultural politics. They give life to the morbid predictions encoded in official and semiofficial surveillance stats.

The first AIDS cases reverberate with a dreaded shock of realization. For example, Angela, a health care worker from PG, related this account:

They say a man shot himself when his doctor told him he had AIDS. This man was known to have a lot of money; he had a job with the Ministry of Works. And because women like a man with a lot of money they say he probably had sex with many women. He was the wild type. People's names came up. People you wouldn't expect. They loved the cash. One woman was a bartender-waitress at a local disco. The owner came to

W O R K

me and asked me if he should fire her. I told him about how
HIV is transmitted. The thing died down. She kept her job.

The circulation of men and money within a region may be a
good predictor of HIV transmission routes. Once infected, sexually
active men who do not use condoms may transmit HIV as they travel
through the country and take breaks between building roads, string-
ing phone and electric lines, transporting goods or working agricul-
tural fields. Until such men have direct empirical proof that they and
the ones they care about are truly in danger of HIV infection, that is,
until they see people getting sick, they seem to dismiss the threat. HIV
thrives on such rash dismissals—viral originals can hide out for years
in healthy hosts while their actively replicating likenesses flow from
one human to another with every opportunity. By the time the originals blow their cover, wasting the host, they may have already made
new hosts of several others. By the time imprudent men have the kind
of proof they want, the surreptitious and changeable viruses that
cause AIDS may win the survival game.

Many men I spoke to boasted a cavalier attitude about AIDS.
Boasting may have been undercut by anxiety and embarrassment, but
that didn't make it any easier to speak seriously about sexual risk
reduction.

One day as I was sitting in the health post office where Angela
worked, three men on a break from work stopped in to chat. When
I brought up the subject, they said that they didn't believe that AIDS
exists. They said—and I can only take this kind of statement as one
designed to be provocative and confusing—that AIDS is something
made up to make people have sex. A man needs to always have more
than one woman, one explained. After all, you can't eat rice and beans
all the time. Another added pointedly that if he gets it, he's got eight
years to enjoy himself and give it to everybody (another perversely
provocative statement, this time betraying an accurate knowledge of
the disease). Someone added that in Guatemala, if they find out

somebody's got AIDS, they shoot him, because he can't give it to any-body from the ground. (Angela interjected that they shoot people in Guatemala for anything. She knows of two young boys who got caught with drugs over there and never returned. One man added that if they catch you with marijuana in Guatemala, they shoot you.) When I asked about condoms, one man complained that they come right off when you juke, that he never has used one, and that they are just not natural. Another claims that only white bati-man (gays) get it. In response to my description of the heterosexual pattern of HIV transmission in Africa, this man declared that if AIDS is in Africa, the white man brought it there. Finally one said that he thinks of sex on an average of thirty-eight times a day, sometimes a hundred times in one day, every time a girl passes by. All three jokingly agreed.

In March, I attended the annual Garifuna Convention in the central coastal town of Dangriga. In a panel discussion on health is-sues, a nurse practitioner told me that there had been five AIDS deaths in that town, four men and one woman, and that these had probably infected over a hundred people out there, although she said they didn't know whom. She said that probably because of the AIDS scare, STD rates are down. However, teen pregnancies are up, starting as young as age twelve, indicating the use of a male risk-reduction strategy that relies on choosing to have sex with younger and younger girls in the hope of avoiding infection.

Most women I talked to did not use condoms with their sex partners. I talked to one woman in her twenties about why she didn't. She was from Orange Walk, a town near the northern border with Mexico, also called Rambo Town for its level of gun violence. When I met her, she was working in Belize City as a domestic in a bed and breakfast. To support her point of view on condoms, she told me the story of a jealous wife who put pepper in her husband's condom, and when he slept with his sweetheart, she ended up having to get a hysterectomy in Merida (on the Mexican side of the border). This seemed particularly galling to the woman with whom I spoke, as her usual risk-reduction strategy was to only have sex with married men with kids, ignoring her mother's advice to "keep what you have between your feet!" She also told me about her brother's wife's brother who had AIDS in the United States. He came back to Orange Walk to marry the woman who once had a son by him in order to legitimize his son's inheritance. Then he went back to the United States. He was gay.

The man hired as the new national AIDS coordinator had expertise in STD contact tracing for the British military. He told me about a Belizean woman who was having sex with her HIV-positive boyfriend without condoms because he doesn't like them. The couple had broken up at some point, and each took another partner. Then they got back together again. The woman says she can't imagine having sex with condoms for the rest of his life.

Dogs and Monkeys

At the panel on health issues at the Garifuna Convention, a nurse reported a measles outbreak in Guatemala with forty cases in Belize. She said they were immunizing the migrant workers who had come to Dangriga to work in the banana and citrus industries. But over the past five years, people had become increasingly concerned about the safety of needles. Needles were being reused without boiling between patients. Parents deliberately kept their children from school on vaccination days.

Public health facts, like the importance of immunizing one's child against the measles, are suspect. Yes, maybe it is good to prevent your child from getting measles, but what if it means "accidentally" giving your child HIV? These fears are plausible. They arise from a healthy skepticism: Medical care is not always the best when it is given to poor people, and sometimes it is downright dangerous. Forces of inequality shape health care as they shape all public institutions. They also fuel fact-resistant politics. When Nurse Peters mentions flatly that the

U.S. government sent two men with AIDS home to Belize, what sentiment does her professionalism mask? Statements by those who don't have a professional stake may be more straightforward, or outrageous, depending on your perspective. Consider this conversation among women at the side of an open-air roadhouse beer joint in PG. Following a lead, I had come to interview the bar owner about sexual risk:

■ Woman bar owner: That thing [AIDS] has been here since the beginning of time. It come from dogs, American women up there having sex with dogs, they catch it from them. Dogs. Here you don't let dogs in the house, they stay outside, cats too.

Woman farmer: I heard it comes from those people in Africa who go to the forest and do things with monkeys. Those monkeys have it and give it to the people.

Woman bar owner (roaring with laughter): A woman up there had sex with a dog and she gave it to her man. That's how it got started!

The bar owner's claims may be interpreted as an ignorant denial of the reality of AIDS as a disease, but that would be a mistake. Her claims are part of a battle that is more about racist politics than about disease. She fights one racist fiction with another. In contrast, the farmer refers uncritically to the widespread monkey theory, a so-called scientific theory weakly supported by evidence. Nevertheless, the putative sexual connection between African monkeys and humans fuels a destructive racist dialogue about the origins of AIDS. Based on the work of Cantwell (1988, 1993), Fiske (1994, 214) explains: [3]

The "green monkey theory" was proposed in the early 1900s by a number of scientists, some of whom worked at Fort Detrick, and may well be a piece of disinformation as clever as anything the Soviets ever produced. It was immensely offensive to African Americans because it assumed sexual contact between Africans and monkeys; usually this assumption was implicit, but this was not always the case: some scientists proposed what Tom Curtis calls "the kinky-African-sex-theory" of a "bizarre sexual practice in which, to heighten sexual arousal, male and female members bordering the large lakes of Central Africa introduce monkey blood into their pubic areas, thighs and backs."[4] Even the more oblique versions of the theory would have their effectiveness enhanced by their resonance with the white animalization and hypersexualization of Black people; they kept alive a history at least stretching back to 1781 and Thomas Jefferson's *Notes on the State of Virginia*. Here, one of the founding fathers described a hierarchy of beauty and sexual desire in which the lust of the Black man for the white woman was as natural as that which the Black woman aroused in the orangutan. Cantwell's research, however, argues too, that the theory that AIDS spread from Africa to the United States, instead of vice versa, cannot explain why a Black heterosexual disease in Africa (almost none of the millions of whites living there have contracted it) could have become a white homosexual disease in the United States. The disease, he concludes, can only have had dual, and almost simultaneous, origins, each aimed at a different population.

In 1990, when people in Belize were thinking about AIDS, they may have been thinking seriously about the deadly viral disease, but they were probably also thinking, "What sick racist crap are they going to try and dump on us now?" The producers of the monkey theory have responsibility for the effects of disseminating this nexus of images. The theory increases tensions between blacks and whites, throwing into question more balanced and useful information and perhaps contributing to an increase in HIV risk among those who resent and resist racial bias paraded as science.[5]

Walking down the road one day alongside a PG townsman in a

wheelchair, another townsman saw us and joked about how he'd better be careful because gringos pass on AIDS. Some joke.

The Outhouse

Racist politics and feigned insouciance may be ways for displacing real fears. Indeed, many people in Belize 1990 were alarmed about AIDS. Poorly informed about modes of transmission, some were terrified by those living with HIV and the bodies of those who had died of AIDS. Hospitals weren't yet diagnosing HIV and AIDS. Angela told me about a case in which the hospital in PG learned only after a man died that he was HIV-infected. The test results returned afterward. They hadn't known what he died from.

The first men, women, and children to die of AIDS in Belize suffered the fears of their friends, families, and caretakers:

■ Nurse Peters of the STD clinic in Belize City told me that they say the cook at the Luxor Restaurant had sex with 140 men. A single mother, she cooked in the day and worked sex at night. The owner, an acquaintance of Nurse Peters, felt that it wasn't any of her business what the woman did at night. But when the fact that she had AIDS came out, she felt badly that someone with AIDS was cooking in her restaurant, and closed it down. It reopened later with new owners. The cook died in the isolation wards of the Belmopan hospital.

■ A woman in Dangriga told me about a pregnant woman with AIDS who was in the hospital there. They put her on the end of a ward where no one goes. They say she has a lot of sex partners and one boyfriend who is HIV-positive.

■ I met a North American ethnobotanist searching for AIDS cures. On a break from the field he was dancing at an upscale Belize City disco. He told me that the woman in the house he stayed in had AIDS;

her symptom was wasting. Despite the fact that there is no epidemio-logical evidence that mosquitoes can transmit AIDS, this man reported that he was scared because there were lots of mosquitoes in the house, and he was covered with blood. He'd also heard about four or five cases of AIDS in PG. One was a young girl who was infected in Los Angeles and came back to die. Her mother burned copal on her shoulders and prayed.[6]

■　　The woman from Orange Walk who told me the pepper in the condom story, also told me about a young boy with AIDS. His mother shut him up in a secluded room day after day until he died. She said that she'd read about it in *The Reporter* the previous year.

■　　The director general of the Red Cross in Belize City told me about the case of an HIV-positive man discharged from the hospital. His family had pushed him into an outhouse and burned all his clothes. The man died.

The work wrought by this virus on the human form sometimes evokes awful responses. Through the compassionate application of scientific knowledge regarding the ways that HIV is most probably transmitted, eventually people will learn that, except where there are breaks in the skin exposing blood, those who are HIV-positive can be touched without fear of infection. As locals join the ranks of foreign ghosts, as the phenomenal world of direct sensory experience catches up with global networks, Belizeans will begin to readjust their acts and their arguments.

4 / Prostitution South

AIDS in Belize 1990 is a story of sex, money, and travel. There was no significant level of intravenous drug use. Crack-cocaine was nipping at the edges, but alcohol and marijuana continued to be the most popular choices. Although each of these substances may decrease the likelihood of sexual risk reduction, none are directly implicated in transmission. The blood supply was supposedly safe. It was a good time for the government to make AIDS prevention a priority. The epidemic still hadn't hit hard. If prevention is effective, maybe it never would.

I thought it would be useful to focus on conditions that put masses of people at risk, rather than focus on the individual (the should-I-or shouldn't-I-use-a-condom dilemmas). I thought about how human populations move HIV from one continent to another, all those sexually active bodies leaping oceans for work and vacation in predictable ways. What happens when transnational circuits of power, pleasure, and infection link up with local, and as yet uninfected, sexual networks?

This was a good plan, and in small countries there is a greater chance that an ethnographer's institutional interventions might actually have an effect. I believe that this turned out to be the case in Belize. Of course, knowing that you can have an impact is different from predicting what the nature of that impact will be. Even in small countries, the complicated politics of intervention reduce the

WORK

predictability of institutional response. Once you set something in motion, you lose whatever control you thought you had.

Transmission Circuits

Peace and the mighty U.S. dollar draw people in to Belize from surrounding Spanish-speaking countries. As the STD clinic records indicate, fear of HIV among migrants, immigrants, and refugees may not be totally unwarranted. But focusing on them to the exclusion of other categories of mobile persons is a way of avoiding discussion about one's own citizens and benefactors. Projecting fear onto others is a form of denial as likely to overtake institutions as individuals.

Foreigners are always moving through Belize: There are tourists and sailors; people in business and government; military personnel from Britain, Nepal, and the United States; Belizean soldiers who leave on missions to strategic ports;[1] Belizean civilians who work in the United States and come back to visit or retire.[2] These transnational flows doubtless include persons from areas of high HIV seroprevalence, many of whom gladly support Belize's thriving sex industry and many of whom find nonprofessional sex partners.

Making the case that conditions for large-scale HIV transmission exist is not enough to induce a commitment to nationwide AIDS prevention programs, however. There are active barriers to instituting prevention. The Catholic Church, for example, provides the financial backbone of social services nationally, particularly education. Where church doctrine contradicts basic tenets of AIDS prevention, as in discussions of homosexuality and condoms, it is not unusual for health professionals to capitulate to the church. The people's representatives in government provide another example. Many think they are there to encourage industry and national (military) security above all else. There are rich incentives to ignore AIDS. Above all is an institutional will to ignorance. Using my preliminary research as a point of departure, I had hoped to tear a hole in the masks. Given my questions, constraints and goals, prostitution provided the most accessible sites to focus my inquiries.

The British VD Doc

I went to the largest base of the British forces, on the road west of town, just past the bar where the owner told me the story about women fucking dogs. I had an appointment with the man they call VD doc, who was actually a med tech. At last count (1988), he said there were twelve HIV infections among the soldiers. (But as the British do not test recruits, a vast area of uncertainty exists, I added.) The troops were taking six-month turns in Belize. They were tested only if they came into the clinic about some other STD or if they were worried. VD doc said that AIDS was not high risk in Belize, so the soldiers didn't have to worry. But did the people here have to worry about the soldiers, I asked? Perhaps they were coming from areas of high HIV prevalence, Edinburgh, for example, a city with a high AIDS rate associated with injecting drug use. Well, he said, there weren't many soldiers from Edinburgh, and most of them were married anyway. What happens to soldiers who were infected with HIV, I asked. They send them away to a special hospital in Britain. What happens if their local sex partners become infected with HIV, I wanted to know. It was clear that he had never considered this.

We discussed only the hetero sex industry servicing the soldiers. Not much was going on in Punta Gorda, he says—a few Guatemalan prostitutes charged twenty dollars for sex behind the wall of a local disco recently. He pulled out a photo album. The prostitutes who worked the whorehouse in Belize City are under strict scrutiny: He waved his hand over portraits of young women inscribed with personal data by a careful bureaucratic hand. (The soldiers went to Belize City and the tourist islands for R&R.) Once he watched as a local Creole girl tried to sneak into the whorehouse; the bouncer told her to get out or pay the house cut. The girls inside were checked once a

WORK

week by a civilian doctor. If a soldier came down with something, they pointed to someone in the photo album. The girls had to insist on condoms. They got two warnings and were out after the third incident. What about men who had sex with men, I asked? That was illegal, he told me, just like drug injecting.[3]

Rubie's

The first I'd heard of it was in a newspaper article about killing fields: Imaginations ran wild when a fetus was found buried there. This was followed by another newspaper article about the woman who admitted that the fetus was hers. She explained that she'd had a miscarriage, not an abortion; she was put in jail anyway. When the whorehouse was in downtown Belize City, it used to be called the Crossroads. In 1990 the illegal, quasi-official whorehouse servicing British soldiers was out on the highway. In addition to soldiers, men of all social classes were said to patronize it.

One rainy Sunday night, a friend arranged for me to interview Juan, the whorehouse owner. Not much was happening inside. We had some drinks in the row of booths dividing lounge from dance floor. No one danced to the jukebox. A long bar ran down one side of the dark and cavernous building. There were more girls than customers, mostly Gurkha soldiers in the British forces. (A woman I know in PG told me why professional women prefer Gurkhas: If a girl takes a black man, she don't take no other that night. If a girl takes a Gurkha, he just shake shakes his tail once or twice like a duck.) The well-dressed girls looked charming and healthy. When it was time to have sex, a couple would link arms and disappear down the back hallway. Then the girl would come back out to the cash register and return to the back again.

We went into Juan's back office. He explained that three-quarters of his clients are British soldiers—"limeys" as they're called in Belize.

The workers come from Honduras, El Salvador, Mexico, and Nicaragua. (He listed all the neighboring countries except Guatemala, whose territorial claims serve as the official reason for the limey soldiers' being there.) The girls report to the army as soon as they arrive. An allied army service organization, the STD doctor, military police, army intelligence, and the secret service are responsible for political and medical surveillance. First, they get the girls drunk and ask some questions. This is followed by an interview, a photograph, and a medical check for AIDS, syphilis, gonorrhea, and chlamydia. In addition to their regular Thursday 6 P.M. checkups, AIDS tests are repeated every three months and syphilis tests every two. Everything is done to assure that the workers are clean. Juan boasts that the army gives him the latest, strongest, and most expensive antibiotics for the girls free. Taking the medicine is mandatory.

I asked how he came to own the whorehouse. He said that he learned to take care of guests at a downtown hotel where he tended bar. He learned how to spot who wants what at the hotel and how to make tips off tourists. Familiarity with the business led to financial backing—his first break. He spoke to girls at other whorehouses. The owners roughed girls up quite a lot. Over here, he told them, the owner would be good to them. They agreed: When he was ready, they would move. He told them how they might even get married to limeys and go live over in England or Germany. He said he knew of three or four who actually did get married, although the army discouraged the practice.

Juan has thirty-two girls. He had only eight rooms when he started, and now he has twenty-five, eight on San Pedro and two on Cay Caulker (two popular resort islands). I offer package deals, he said: A person comes in and wants a companion, I fly her in and out. I link up with people every day. Right now someone wants five girls for three days in Placencia (a coastal fishing village that is popular with tourists and soldiers). Pandering is part of the regular services provided to men traveling alone on business; the management lets them know girls are available.

As for fees, Juan said that there's a standard price for Belizean and British army clients. Short time is a half hour for $40 Bz, straight thing ($40 Bz = $20 U.S.). Ten to use the room and $30 for the girl. Other than the room fee, everything they make is for them. If the person wants an hour, the room price is $15. The girl takes the man to the room, gets the money and brings it up front to the cashier, and gets a ticket with name and price. Then the doorman gets the ticket. If the girls don't bring them out, the doorman knocks on the door at the right time. This provides protection if people take advantage or if there are fights or complaints.

There's often a language problem in the initial negotiations, and a newcomer might not know what to expect. But every room had condoms, and the girls were required to use them with soldiers. If a soldier gets a sexually transmitted disease and identifies a particular girl from among the surveillance photos in the clinic on base, the girl is held responsible for failure to use a condom. First she gets a warning, the second warning comes with a fine of $100–$200, and the third time the girl is out. With other kinds of customers, it's up to the customer. Most use condoms, but there are plenty Belizeans and Americans who refused. Local girls, the free-lancers, are who caused this business to be successful. If the British army had thirty gonorrhea cases, twenty-nine would be traced to the street.

I asked how he found girls. He explained: They have a communication network. I only went two times looking for girls. A friend in Honduras solicited for me in Puerto Cortez, a transcontinental port town. The girls crossed the border illegally, and I'd pick them up at a certain point and bring them in. They were trained by the manager, a pro herself. I asked why he hires Spanish and not Belizean girls. He says that he has no control over Belizean girls. Medical doctors' checkups are compulsory, and if they're put off sex they have to be put off totally. A Belizean girl can go home, and I don't know if she takes her medication or not. And when he prescribes that expensive antibiotic cyproxin for gonorrhea, we have to follow it up with tetracycline: We give them water and they drink it down out in front.

Is there something about race that makes the limeys think the Spanish are more exotic than the local black Creole women? It varies, some limeys do have a thing for black girls. But, he says, the girls available out there are hustlers, and in a short time the men realize why the army doesn't want them to have sex with them. They get VD. The girls out there don't know what a doctor is. Back in 1985, a politician named Fred Smith started a campaign against gonorrhea and some other STD. The rates had gotten so out of hand (some three hundred cases), that the army put Belize City out of bounds. They sent policemen around to where the girls would be. The policemen brought the girls in to get injections. They forced them to be treated. It's easy to find them at the Balcony, the Pub, the Bellevue. Fred Smith monitored the girls, identified each one, but some would only come out on weekends and some had no address.

What about male prostitutes, I asked. Six or seven guys were working the Balcony, but that was banned. They were also banned from the Pub. They came up here to solicit soldiers. I feel pity for bati-men, but I wouldn't allow them to hail me on the street. Same little bunch of guys, five or six of them, they called me and said it was a free country. I had the cops beat them up. I've got to think of my reputation. I didn't want to be known as having girls and guys available.

How long do girls usually stay, I asked. It depends on the management and the girl. I control them like family. They don't use drugs, don't get drunk, don't steal money, and don't fight with other girls. Sometimes there's jealousy over a client and there's a fight with a knife or ice pick. Last thing I want is one of the girls to get killed.

They make an average of between $500 and $1,000 Bz a week (=$250–$500 US).[4] They come green from little villages. They've never done this in their country. They range from sixteen to twenty-five years old. They may have done this before, but not as professionals. In their countries, they can work in a shoe store for practically nothing. If they have a child, the fathers abandoned them, there are no good jobs, they're forced to hustle. When they go home for vacation, every day twenty-five other girls would say to them "Get me to Belize." Some are educated. One is a Honduran architect who's been here eight months. There are three sisters who will open a supermarket.

Blow jobs? Blow jobs are seventy-five dollars for two to three minutes. Belizeans have never . . . fishermen on San Pedro and Cay Caulker have only dreamt about blow jobs. If you ask for a blow job in Orange Walk, they'll think you're crazy. This whorehouse is modern and sophisticated. Anal sex . . . I wouldn't know about, but it's not that unusual to charge a hundred dollars per customer.

My business is successful only if they don't get sick: Getting sick means losing money. Then he pulled out a bunch of pharmaceuticals from his desk drawer, explaining about compulsory treatment. The interview ended shortly after that, when all the lights went out.

The Balcony

The new man hired to coordinate AIDS intervention and surveillance in the country and I had overlapping goals, so I suggested we do some

A similar version of "The Balcony" appeared earlier in *Canadian Folklore canadien,* 15(1): 109–17, and is reprinted here by permission.

fieldwork together. We set a date to meet at the Balcony on Thirsty Thursday. I was anxious about going alone, so I went to his office the morning we were to meet to remind him of our appointment. When he began apologizing for not showing up, I suspected he had no intention of coming. But I did not change my plan, even though I knew the time he'd proposed, 9 P.M., was way too early. I wore the unsexiest tropical clothing I could find and asked some of my middle-class white Creole friends to drop me off—they wouldn't think of hanging out in the place. They wanted to know about what I was doing, so I told them I needed to check out the prostitution scene, and they were quite taken aback that I thought that what was going on there was prostitution. "Those are Belizean women who go there. Belizean women aren't prostitutes. They're just out for a good time, some free drinks, you know, partying." Hmmm, I thought, I'd been there before and it sure looked like prostitution to me, taking note of the gap between our perceptions. (I was operating with the general definition that prostitution is a form of exchange involving sex and money or other goods.)

Walking upstairs to confront the two bouncers at the door, who said something like, "Hey lady, do you know this is Belize?" I said, with a bravura I did not really feel, that "yes, thank you, I know where the fuck I am." It was pretty empty. The white soldiers, mostly boys still wet behind the ears, were bunched up out on the balcony, and inside, not far from the bar. The television was tuned to CNN, and if I remember right, it was something about Michael Jackson visiting the Bushes in the White House and Israeli children getting wrapped up in chemical weapons suits in preparation for Iraqi attacks. A few black Creole women and black and white Creole men sat at the bar watching. On the balcony, a few black Creole women and one black Creole man were entertaining limeys with conversation, laughter, and seductive gestures. I got a beer and sat down at a table where I had a good view of everything, and watched and waited. Everyone was watching and waiting; as I say, it was early.

The women, dressed up and looking pretty, began to stake out positions at the tables against the wall. The band started setting up. This AIDS coordinator fellow would be a no-show for sure, I thought. People started to wonder what I was doing there alone. More people eventually showed up, and by the time the band started playing, the place was jumping. Stanley, a black man, was the most boisterously sexual person in the place. The life of the party, he moved round and round, teasing the soldiers, enlivening the subtext of homoeroticism among them, getting the women worked up, and being friendly to me, for which I was grateful. The Chinese owners, flanked by three black Creole, one Latina, and one Chinese woman, sat as still as statues along the wall opposite me, also watching the scene.

The limeys started getting drunker, louder, and more integrated. The women who'd staked out positions at the tables earlier were now squeezed in by men. The dance floor became the focus. I began training my attention on the conditions that would shape the enactment of risk, more particularly, the sexual and ethnic identities of the people, the geography and rhythm of activities, and the sexualization of social interaction. I danced with a pimp who had been sending over beers I could not refuse. He wasn't too sticky, though, and I was on my own again, when I struck up a conversation with a woman, a soldier in the Belize Defense Forces, who came from Punta Gorda. She introduced me to another older woman, who seemed to be there looking out for the younger women. I told them what I was doing there. One of them said, "Oh, you're the public health lady!" Belize is a small country. It happened that her cousin was the secretary of the man who was supposed to meet me there, and they had spoken about me.

By midnight, the bar scene was really hopping. Stanley was doing some wild maneuvers with a black Creole woman on the dance floor, pretending to have sex with her, acting out the bisexual possibilities for the limeys, who were now mostly paired off with local women.

Other Belizean locals started coming out, and even some men from the Belize Defense Forces, who weren't supposed to frequent this place, showed up. The crowd was loosening up, intermingling. The sex trade was by now effectively indistinguishable from the regular night life of the city.

Stigma, Social Organization, and Risk

The Latina women in the whorehouse and the Belizean Creole women in the bars have different strategies for managing the stigma of prostitution. Leaving their personal lives behind, the Latinas become border-crossing sex professionals whose contacts are limited to whorehouse personnel and customers. These illegal aliens enter the country with a nod, a wink, and an interrogation. They shed the stigma of sex work when they depart, crossing back into their lives with hard-won financial reserves. That's how I would summarize Juan's version of the story anyway.

In contrast, Belizean Creole women who service soldiers draw them into their personal lives. Refusing professional identity, they neutralize the stigma associated with prostitution. Their work circuit is embedded in the night life of the city—different nights, different bars. They expect their limey sex partners to provide for them materially, just as Belizean boyfriends and husbands are expected to do. Money is just part of the regular deal. Ask anyone.

Belizeans generally seemed complicit in this charade, because they sure don't want to think that their beautiful, black, and independent Creole mothers, sisters, cousins, and aunts are whoring for the fucking limeys. . . . None of this makes much difference, of course, unless the virus seeps in.[5] Viruses have DNA, but no brain. They might not even be animals. They're just replicating machines flowing from one wet orifice to another. We give them life by opening ourselves up to each other. Unfortunately, HIV thrives on the foibles of friendship, passion, and love.

69

When heterosexuals just meet and, within a few hours, mutually consent to engage in casual sex, a woman wouldn't want or expect to be considered a prostitute, nor the man someone's customer. For many, the image of condoms is fused to this something out there that you do not want to be confused with, a whore, a trick. This may explain why condoms are less likely to be used in casual, nonprofessional sex than in professional sex.[6]

I thought about the contrast between nonprofessional and professional sexual risk because of what I'd learned from prostitutes in Chicago. It was common to hear them say that they had always used condoms with tricks but never with lovers. Condoms marked the boundary that separated the streets from their personal lives, a symbolic maneuver that gave them room to be themselves. But some had boyfriends who shot dope, and maybe they didn't always use clean needles. For these women, the danger of HIV came from the one they loved, not the many they serviced.

The high rates of gonorrhea in Belize indicate that unprotected sex is not uncommon.[7] If women who worked the Balcony did not define their sex acts with multiple partners of casual acquaintance for money or goods as prostitution, a professional context in which condoms are more likely to be part of the sexual code, then they would need to create the alternative scenario—romantic love. And unfortunately, condoms may not be a helpful prop. The women who worked sex out of the bars were also at risk due to a lack of AIDS education and access to free condoms. As far as I could determine, there had been no outreach to these women. Their risk was obscured by the general sense that what was going on in the bars and hotels between Creole women and limey soldiers was just ordinary, good-time hetero sex, the Belizean national pastime.[8] This is yet another version of the North American denial script about being safe if one was not this, that, or the other—never mind your behavior.

The Politics of Intervention

After collecting and analyzing the data, I wrote a report to the Ministry of Health that sketched out transnational forces that could be associated with HIV transmission patterns in Belize. I handed it out to all the officials and quasi-officials involved in AIDS prevention and care. The aim of the report was to identify possible outreach targets, with a focus on prostitution. It described how the unnamed whorehouse of obvious identity was one of the safest places to engage in sex with someone whom you did not know well. Risk reduction in the form of condom use was an integral part of the professional code. Although the threat of sanction lay unfairly with the women, mandatory condom use protected both Latina workers and their soldier tricks.

Seizing on the differences between prostitution in whorehouses and the quasi-prostitution taking place in bars, the report attempted to facilitate institutional change in two ways. First, it provided information that could be used to help design AIDS outreach efforts, if the government was ready to do so. It suggested that providing information and condoms to the local women who played or worked in the Belize City bars would be an appropriate starting point. Second, the report suggested that if Belizeans are at risk as a result of unprotected sexual contact with British troops, perhaps this factor should enter into negotiations between Belize and British governments. If transmission between soldiers and local women occurs, should the British government assume some responsibility for care and prevention? How many cases would it take? Given the general lack of testing, how would the governments know how many cases there were? I thought it was worth raising these questions, although I suspected that those who benefited from the British military presence would resist risking troop withdrawal in order to protect the health of what they might perceive as a few poor women.

WORK

Over the next few months, the report generated interest among officials and researchers. I presented it publicly on a panel with government health and education officials and felt that I played a role in triggering a new level of public awareness and accountability.[9] This was only one side of the story, however. I am not so proud of the other side. After I wrote the report, I made a trip to the States to mark my passage from researcher to ordinary traveler. Not long after my return to Belize, I ran into Juan in the Belize City bank. He said only that he was sorry that he ever met me and that Rubie's was closed. I was shocked and dismayed. As far as I could find out, the British military responded fairly swiftly to the report with an action that precisely contradicted its public health implications: They had declared Juan's whorehouse off limits to soldiers. If my hypothesis is correct, this would have shifted the soldier tricks away from the relative safety of a whorehouse with mandatory condom use and toward the higher risk of the unregulated bars, thereby intensifying the risk of HIV transmission of the sex workers of their host country as well as of their own soldiers.

The report accomplished the exact opposite of my intent. I can only speculate that for the British military, public image was more important than public health; in other words, let's brush these annoying matters under the carpet for a while so the church can go on pretending not to notice the whorehouse is there. What is confusing to me is that I didn't really say anything about the place that everyone didn't already know. The existence and function of the whorehouse was common knowledge, but officially it did not exist. My mistake was translating common knowledge into official discourse. In effect then, my mission was doomed before it started. My idealism led me to rely on the unrealistic assumption that governments act for the good of the people. My idealism blinded me to the power of hypocrisy.[10]

Frankly, the whole intervention reminds me of the Chicken Drop: The Chicken Drop is a game of chance. A man keeps a chicken in a dark box. When the people gather round, he suddenly shakes the box, dumping the chicken out on a floor. The floor is drawn with numbered boxes. When the chicken shits on one of the numbers, winning bets collect.

Applied anthropology is a chancy business. When ethnographers act beyond the usual sphere of academic influence and use knowledge to trigger change, they have a responsibility to attend the political force field and act with caution. In the real world of human interaction, predictive power is limited (you can never tell into which box the chicken will shit). My intervention failed if measured by my intention. However, the failure told me more about the forces at play than all the steadfast data collection and analysis that preceded it. The trick is to initiate change without causing harm.

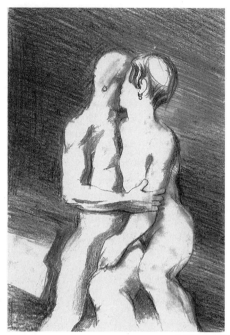

PART II *Escape*

Stepping in
and out
of fragrant beds
and sweating
in fabulous bath
houses, ranks
among today's
great
comedies,
especially
if you cop
a fix before
going in
and out.
Save me
the cotton,
thanks! Death smiles,
it has
a sense
of humor.

— *C. Jason Dotson*

5 / Death Rite

They Buried Her Ten Feet Deep

A health care worker once told me about a twenty-two-year-old Garifuna woman who died of AIDS. *She had left PG for Dangriga to live with a man and their children. She came back to PG with* AIDS. *Or so they thought, as she suffered wasting and difficult breathing. It was kind of a hush-hush thing. Few came to the wake. People were afraid to eat in the house. They buried her ten feet deep.*

Eventually AIDS soaks into all arenas of social life. In 1990 Belize there was still much fear and uncertainty associated with the bodies of the few Garifuna persons who died of AIDS. Families were apparently unprepared to stage the full rites under those circumstances. But someday the passage of some of those who have died of AIDS may also be honored by drumbeat and song. In that spirit, I offer this account.

Double Ninth Night in Barranco

They say that the vessels carrying men, women, and children kidnapped from Africa for America's slave trade foundered off the coast of Honduras before ever reaching shore. Many swam to safety, survived, and married into Arawak Indian families. Their descendants live today along the coast divided by the national boundaries of

Nicaragua, Belize, Guatemala, and Honduras. "We are the only African people in the new world who never experienced slavery," said a Garifuna elder in Belize.

Except perhaps for regular travel between the Caribbean coast and the large Garifuna communities in the HIV epicenters of Los Angeles and New York, the Garifuna are no more or less at risk of AIDS than the Creoles, Mayan, East Indians, Spanish, Chinese, or Anglo-American people who live in Belize. I was drawn to participate more directly in Garifuna culture by the strength and coherence of their ritual practices. I wondered how AIDS—as a master signifier—would collide with a traditional symbol system that uses pleasure to defend against pain.

Sex is the best protection against Death, or so I interpret the use of sexual imagery in Garifuna wakes, called ninth nights or *beluria*. According to tradition (when families have the resources, skills, and desire to follow it), the ninth night after someone dies, family and friends gather in from homes along the Caribbean coast (see Kerns 1997). They come to dance and drum and sing and talk and laugh and eat to mark the deceased's crossing out of the familiar world. In this way, Death is sent on its merry way, and the circle of mourners are seduced away from grief. The event I describe here took place in the small Garifuna fishing village of Barranco, an hour or so by motorized dory down the coast from Punta Gorda. This ninth night was unusual in that two families put their resources together and had a double rite. The two deceased in question had died some time before, one about three weeks before the other. There was only one corpse, as one had died and was buried in the States.

People seemed to anticipate ninth nights as they might anticipate a party, although it takes a great deal of work and money to organize. I interpret the strong festive dimension of wakes as a stubborn expression of joy in the face of loss. The fire of survival burns in the drumbeat, in the dancers' whirls, in the anger of song. Blood pulses, the senses rejoice. The delicious rice pudding, cassava bread, and beans that the women prepared and served with sweetened coffee and rum mark the occasion's importance. By fulfilling a traditional set of expectations, the ritual restores a sense of order to the void created by the death of a loved one. It eases pain and sorrow and confirms the generosity and continuity of kinship.

The ritual space for this ninth night consisted of three wooden buildings and the space alongside: one small house held the single coffin with altar and benches; a larger house with a tin-roofed porch constructed for this night held a second altar and set of benches; a third little kitchen building sat behind. Once a day during the preceding week of preparation, a group of women had gathered each twilight to pray at the altars. Now that the ninth night event was beginning, dancers and conga drummers filled the open area alongside the larger house. The focus of ritual action kept alternating between indoor New Testament prayer and outdoor Garifuna dance. Most participants stayed outside. A muted phase of Catholic prayer would bring the mourners' attention through the candle-lit windows to those seated within. Then the joyful sounds of an intact African tradition would become the dominant presence. Male drummers, well-supplied with rum and tobacco, kept the beat strong and unified, energizing the dancers. After midnight, a full meal with coffee was served. The meal was followed by rum, crème de menthe and cigarettes for all. Supplies were limited.

The dance phase lengthened and intensified after the meal. People stood in a wide circle around the drummers. The action became focused on the dancers who jumped inside the circle one or two at a time, usually a woman and man, sometimes two couples. One man might tap another man on the shoulder, one woman might tap another woman to indicate that it was time to switch partners. Young and old danced together. Dancers wound their buttocks in motions mimicking intercourse, a pleasure-inducing practice refined through the centuries to incite the eye to imagine the touch. But no touch was allowed. If a male dancer got a bit fresh and came too close, his partner would push him back or huff out of the circle. Even a really old woman got in the circle. She cast off her usual stoop to display a mastery of her gender's pleasure and her culture's lifeline. Vibrant sparks beamed from the eyes of the ancient one. Women chanted songs to the drumbeat. They refused to let drummers rest much between songs. Song after Garifuna song came forth. Songs encoded their own breaks, signaling shifts in the dancers' movements. One woman liked to thrust her hips out toward the drummers for emphasis. She practically climbed on their heads and knocked them down at times.

One song was just for women dancers. There were two pieces of wood put on the ground in the middle of the circle. As each woman took her turn, she picked up one of the pieces of wood and hit the other piece with it. The song was about the dead body of a man on a beach, someone explained to me. The women were each taking their turn killing this man because he was a man who liked to beat women. When signaled by a stanza's end, each woman performed her own unique jump out of the circle. The drumming and dancing continued till dawn. As the hours wore on, it sounded as if it were mostly women who kept it going. At dawn, I heard the men's voices again. At about 8 A.M., just as their voices sounded strongly, someone came to tell them it was time to end. After a long sleep, everyone dispersed, reentering their everyday lives renewed.

6 / Losing It

Fugitive Redemption

In big cities like Chicago, many individuals are isolated from families and other community institutions that might help them with economic resources and meaningful rituals in times of trouble. Indeed, isolation may hasten the slide into addiction, a set of psycho-physiological obsessions with their own demanding and often cruel rituals of engagement.

If it weren't for its astonishing power of destruction, drug addiction would attract no special interest. Addiction is a challenge of doubtful reward. Getting trapped requires determination. (Many people throw up a lot trying to get used to heroin, for example.) Successful addicts must learn to market their talents in a local system of organized behaviors, just like everyone else. Becoming adept at thieving, con, or selling sex or dope allows the addict to control the intervals between full syringes. The more adept you are, the more opportunities you have to reign in that fugitive redemption.

This chapter is about two women, an addict and a wife, both raised Catholic in their mid-twenties, both European (or whites in black parlance). One was living off the Latino copping networks on westside Chicago, and one found her way to a southside shelter from rural Illinois. I interviewed them in the field stations of the AIDS intervention project. I call them Boots and Sandy. Their personal histories trace the lay of the land.[1]

Routine

I was pretty surprised when Boots walked into the westside station. It was that Daughters of America look. But the bruised eye and hungry edge tipped me off that she might be a convincing study participant. She introduced herself as Tommy the pimp's new girl, but she was working freelance. She said she gave him money sometimes because she liked him. He pampered his girls and had a formidable reputation. (He was supposed to have killed three people and was wanted in Philadelphia. He tortured some guy who cut off one of his girls' ears.) Boots said that she and Tommy have a lot of fun together.

She shot drugs at least five times a day and had been working sex for three months. She qualified for the study, which meant she would get ten dollars to have her blood drawn and tested, ten dollars for the NIDA surveillance interview, and ten dollars for an ethnographic interview: That's thirty dollars, enough to buy dope. First she explained the bruises: Yesterday, her friend took her to cop. The punk brother of a local gang leader called her friend an asshole. So she said, "Don't call him an asshole." He said, "Shut up, you dirty whore." She slapped him, and he punched her hard twice. It knocked her back five feet, she saw stars, grabbed on to a car, stood there for a second to let everything get back into sight, then turned and walked away.

The surveillance interview provided some crucial details: Born and raised in Cincinnati, she had become a twenty-five-year-old Buddhist with some college experience. She'd had her own apartment for seven months, but she was moving out. She had no children. She first got drunk at nine, first used pot at eleven, first shot up something at twelve, first shot up cocaine at fourteen, heroin at fifteen, and speedballs at twenty-four (a regular just-say-no textbook case). Speedballs (a mixture of heroin and cocaine), were her preferred drug combination. She shot this at least four or five times a day, a habit that cost three hundred dollars a day. She did barbiturates two to six times a week; alcohol about once a week; freebase, methadone, opiates, and tranqs less than four times a month. She'd been in treatment lots of times, mostly detox-residential settings in the suburbs. She always cleaned her needles with bleach and, except with current boyfriends, always used condoms for intercourse. She used condoms when convenient for oral sex (90 percent of her professional activities were oral). She worked seven days a week and serviced 3 to 5 tricks a day. With about half her tricks being regulars, that came to about 150 men in her first three months, 4 of whom she knew were injectors. Her health was excellent, and she was not sure if she was pregnant, she said.

A friend of hers was outside waiting for her in his car. He was a straight-looking ex-cop who worked at some treatment program. It had taken a couple of hours to do the blood and the interviews. I went along with them afterwards to observe. Boots and I walked a few blocks over to a house with two sentries (one of a zillion places around there to cop, she said). The friend followed in the car. Boots walked up to one of the sentries and said, "Two brown and one white." We waited on a stoop a couple of minutes, and he brought her three tiny aluminum foil packages. I think she paid him the whole thirty dollars she made at the field station. We got into the friend's car and drove to buy a needle. Boots went into a two-story building with a really rough-looking character standing out front (older than the sentries who sold her the dope). She came out and said the guy who sells the needles was at the bar. The people inside were charging money for shooting up, even though it wasn't their house. We drove over to the bar, and she went inside, found the guy, bought a sealed needle for $2.50 and got back in the car.

Squeezed between me, stick shift, and ex-cop, Boots reached into her pocket to pull out the cut bottom of an empty beer can and one of the little bottles of bleach the project handed out, which she had refilled with water. She emptied the powder from all three packets into the can bottom, added a little water and heated the mixture with a lighter from below. The car was unsteady. When the dope dissolved, she drew it up and stuck the syringe into the open seam that ran along the top edge of her hand. We made our way across the city to her apartment. She got it into the vein on the second try. As the dope coursed though her bloodstream, there didn't appear to be any significant mood shift. She spoke just as coolly, but her aura changed. I detected what I can only describe as a silent buzz around her face. She said she wasn't high, she was just okay and her stomach ache was gone. She had last shot up at 6 A.M., and it was about 6 P.M. by the time she got that hit. Sometime that night she'd have to go out and trick again to make another buy.

Her apartment looked normal for a twenty-six-year-old middle-class single woman—furniture, artwork, plants. It was in a Polish neighborhood where everybody knows everybody, "Not the right kind of place for Boots," explained her friend on the way over. We'd brought a bunch of empty cartons for her to pack. She was planning on moving in with Tommy the pimp's mother. Her friend drove me back to the station.

Disruption

Sandy left her hometown in rural Illinois with her four- and five-year-old and fifteen dollars. She escaped from her cocaine-crazed husband. She was a refugee in southside Chicago, a place she'd never been, among black people whose images she knew only through television. She got help. The cops put her in touch with people at Human Services, who arranged for her to stay in a woman's shelter. They also promised to get her on Public Aid, and in a few weeks, pay the initial deposit on an apartment (the social safety net at its best). She changed her name so that her husband couldn't trace her. I got her alias and location from George, the outreach worker who stopped by the shelters as part of his regular circuit. On the phone, she said she was extremely frightened about AIDS. Her husband was a cocaine addict who burglarized for a living. He wouldn't let her work. Their home became a shooting gallery (though she didn't use that term). His friends would come around to shoot up, hang out. She said there was always blood everywhere: on the walls, in the sinks, on the towels.

She fit the epidemiological category of sex partner: a person who does not shoot drugs themselves, but who has a sex partner who does. I picked her and her kids up in my car and drove to the station for an interview. She could use the thirty dollars. Sandy occasionally drank alcohol or smoked pot; once she joined her husband on a co-caine binge and didn't like it. While sex with her husband scared her because of AIDS, the blood and needles she saw around the house scared her more. The interview began with Sandy sketching out her situation:

■   I got back with him about a month and a half ago, and he had a couple of jobs for a couple of days here and there. It never lasted long, because he'd start with drugs. He would burglarize and get money. I'd say that I need rent and I need food. I need a shelter over my kids' head, and he didn't want to work, so he would go out and burglarize. Instead of getting money for what he stole, such as copper coiling or burglarizing houses, he would get cocaine in payment for merchandise rather than money. And he would do the cocaine. Approximately two or three weeks after I got back with him, in that month and a half he started shooting. Then I just saw in the three or four weeks that I saw him shoot it, it got way out of hand. There were people coming over constantly, all hours of the day, more and more people. He just got more and more careless and more and more less concerned about anything, but the drug. I just was trying to maintain a certain lifestyle for my kids and trying to change him and it wasn't working. It was getting worse and worse.

He just continues to hang around with these lowlifes and with people that do it. He lived in one house all his life and the same neigh-borhood and knows everybody in that town, practically. He gets rid of one group of creeps and another one comes along. He falls from one group to the next, and they all seem to be doing drugs, and drugs these days is cocaine.

Sandy and her husband only rarely had sex. If they did, it would be straight intercourse; he didn't deserve head, and he didn't like condoms. They did try condoms a couple of times when a neighbor had some. She used spermicide for birth control but didn't always have the money to buy it. A couple of times in the previous weeks her husband asked her to have sex. He said, "What are you afraid of, getting AIDS? She said, "Yes. You might have AIDS and you don't know. I don't want it, I have kids to raise, and I don't want these kids in this world by themselves."

Sandy got several true-false questions on AIDS knowledge wrong on the surveillance interview: whether a positive blood test means the person has AIDS; whether latex condoms effectively protect you from the virus; whether you can get AIDS from a needle sold on the street in a sealed wrapper; whether you can get AIDS from shaking hands, from donating blood or plasma, from eating in a restaurant where a cook has AIDS, or from public toilets; whether cleaning works with bleach is an effective way of killing the virus.

But perhaps her deviations from official knowledge were not as ignorant of the facts as they seemed: Not all scientists agree that HIV alone is responsible for AIDS. Even doctors, insurance companies, and the CDC are sometimes unsure of how to identify the definitive moment a person who is infected with HIV has AIDS. Latex condoms break, slip off, and are refused by many sexually active men and women, even when they are offered in the spirit of mutual protection. There had been rumors going around Chicago that some illegal needle sellers were resealing used needles, but unless you were a diabetic with a doctor's prescription for needles, you had no choice but to buy them on the street. As far as we know, we can't get AIDS from touching HIV in any way other than when our warm body fluids are in direct contact with another human's warm body fluids. But HIV does *not* magically or instantaneously meet its demise on contact with air, as we project researchers and outreach workers were trained to reassuringly reiterate to all the folks. It takes time to die in air, and whether this means minutes or hours depends on the amount and kind of fluid, the concentration of the virus, and the temperature. In concentrations much higher than normally occur outside of the lab, HIV can live for 2.9 days in sewage (Niedringhaus 1990). In refrigerated corpses, the virus has been found to live for up to sixteen and a half days (Douceron et al. 1993). Nor is bleach the foolproof sanitizer we once thought as we handed out all those thousands of little bottles of bleach to injectors. Years later, NIDA pronounced that bleach is better than nothing, but not as good as a clean needle (and in a decrepit march toward progress, some states are legalizing needle exchange programs).[2]

Indeed, we know very little about some very mundane characteristics of HIV, like which cleaning fluid is best to use when cleaning up a spill. The point is that Sandy's incorrect answers reflect both a lack of knowledge and a pragmatic cynicism that puts her mistakes on the side of cautious paranoia. I wonder if our public health messages are too soothing, training public concern on only the most obviously dangerous risks.

Ostensibly designed to control panic, public health messages that inaccurately gloss over unknown and dubious aspects of viral biology may wind up actually inciting panic. This is part of a multilayered phenomenon. Erni (1994) analyzes the way in which medical and media discourse focuses on scientists working toward a cure at the same time they represent AIDS as incurable. He argues that the proliferation of contradictions and instabilities surrounding the notion of an AIDS cure creates a complex phantasmic and paranoid drama that is a crucial carrier of political power (pp. xvi–xvii). His analysis could be applied to discourse on the subject of HIV transmissibility (for example, that you can't get it from kissing because HIV can't live in saliva, but you may be able to get it from "deep kissing" [Altman 1997]).

Sandy's husband had been a heavy drug user for the previous five years, but he had only recently started using needles. Since then he'd been hospitalized three times. She gave him two or three years on the outside before he has a brain hemorrhage or a heart attack. She was firm about giving up on him: "I've tried begging and pleading and fighting and threatening. There's nothing I can do." I asked if she knew of other women who might be in a similar position in her hometown. She said yes, but she didn't talk to them: "Because the men go out, the women stay embarrassed and ashamed and confused, in their apartments, wondering what to do, trying to figure it out. What's going on? Why is it going on? How can I stop it? What can I do? Hiding their money, stuff like that. Hoping that maybe it will stop, but it won't." She suggests a television advertisement targeting women hiding in their houses. It should tell them to take their kids and leave, to just get up and get out. It could say, "Hey! Go get help or stay here and die."

> War is *productive* destructiveness, not only in the sense that it shifts boundaries, defines states, alters the balances of power (*that* we understand)—but in a more profound sense. War creates *the* people. War produces power, individual and collective. War is the cultural property of peoples, a system of signs that we read without much effort because they have become so familiar to us. (Elshtain 1987, 166–67)

Against the backdrop of the short and dramatic postnuclear U.S. television wars is the internal war that grinds depressingly into everyday life. It grinds so slowly that people come to accept war as policy; so plausibly that they even vote for it. I do not believe that the war on drugs is waged for the purpose of helping the citizenry by stopping drug addiction. Without the war on drugs, we would not have this level of addiction and violence in our homes and streets and in the lives of ordinary women like Boots and Sandy. The upheaval in their lives is a result of state-sponsored warfare, evidence of the omnipresence of militarism in human experience (see Cuomo 1996).

Nostalgia

There isn't any one start to a drug history, no one reason why people start taking pleasure in self-destruction. We started the ethnographic interview when Boots was five, because her well-honed therapeutic narrative tied her troubles to her parents' divorce. Boots wasn't doing her homework. She was confused. Her father remarried. She and her stepmother had problems. There was a triangle. Boots got spanked for drinking a beer in the closet when she was seven. When she was eleven, she and her stepsister found a locked box of her father's. They broke into it and found dildos and steam roller (glass) pipes and about a pound of reefer. She lived with her mother in the same neighborhood until her father made it as one of Chicago's top new models and bought an estate. She moved out to the suburbs too, going to junior high and high school out there. Family tensions worsened. Boots started looking for men. She got a job working for a senile pharmacist who would always leave his keys laying around. She was fifteen, and head over heels in love with a guy she met at a gas station (Man 1). Her parents went out of town that summer and she was supposed to move into a girlfriend's house, but instead she joined some friends whose parents had died in a car crash and left them their suburban house. They were making (angel) dust and MDA in the basement.[3] So between that and the pharmacy, by the time her father came back to town she couldn't stand up straight or talk. They put her in the hospital. Three months later they sent her to school-therapy in the Berkshires. Boots was back home outside Chicago for her senior year, then went straight out to work.

Her second love (Man 2) came from a heavy-duty Mafia family.

His father was a doctor, probably the only one who was legit. She lived with Man 2 for four years. All they did was sell cocaine.

■ We had a lot of money. We would take off and fly to Florida and we would just meet some crazy people and you just always needed to find a new place to do cocaine. We wouldn't sleep for days. We would fight. He did this (gesturing to a scar), this was a lot of stitches. We would have crazy fights. It was just a crazy life. We had a lot of money and we were just kids. We went all over and we did whatever we wanted to do. Neither of us worked. We had boats.

Boots moved out after four years and got a job and her own apartment in the city. She was already addicted to heroin. She worked for her stepfather doing property management. She'd travel to all the different buildings every day, stopping here and there to get what she needed. Boots was doing heroin only once a day. She'd do it and go back to work, and no one would know. Heroin was her own little world, her own private rebellion. That lasted about six months. She got into a real ripper fight one night with Man 2, and he did this (gestures to another scar). She was battered from head to toe and had two black eyes. He'd done that to her a couple of times. Boots figured they fought because all the drugs wiped out their mental defenses, so they couldn't defend their feelings. Boots said, "When we got hurt, we hurt back, in the only way, at that time, we knew how. I threw vases at him. He chased me. It's still glass in the wall at this poor little apartment. He chased me around with guns. We had some doozies. It wasn't all the time, but we would go through it once every two or three months." Boots stopped going to work and started doing more and more drugs, but she'd always call her mother, who was there for her no matter what. She called her one morning and she figures that she probably did a lot of Valiums and had passed out while on the phone. Her mother got scared, came and broke down the door of her apartment and took her to the hospital. She was twenty-one by then.

My questions were designed to elicit a chronology of the events that brought her to the present. She suffered loss of memory, she said, and could tell only about the major incidents—those marked out by previous therapists as key stepping-stones in her ongoing narrative, I guessed.

After Boots got out of the hospital from the Valium overdose, she started back in a shooting gallery. Then she met Man 3, who still tracks her down through the neighborhood. "He's forty-one, but he's weird," she said. "He would keep me up all hours of the night and telling what a whore, slut, junkie you are, but then he would never let me go. I love you, I love you. I'll love you to the day I die. I want you in my arms. I have pages, stacks of just love letters he writes. He's the one that gave me the keys to the car." (He had lent her a stolen car, and she went to jail for auto theft. The police thought she ripped off a date and stole the keys. They said all sorts of nasty things. The funny part was, she had seen them on her way to pick up the car and she'd asked, "Would you guys give me a lift, I have to go pick up this car?" "Cross my heart," she said. "I was reading the letter from Man 3 that said here's the keys.")

There was another guy (Man 4) that wanted her to date him all the time. He was a twenty-nine-year-old multimillionaire with a Ferrari Testarossa, a house in California, a condo here, and he could fly wherever he wanted. This guy could have anybody, but he wanted Boots. She called him up the other day, and he said come on by, but as she didn't know where he lived, she said meet me on a corner. He picked her up and did nothing, sat on the (car) telephone, held her, gave her a T-shirt and two hundred dollars. She said, "I've got to go, I thought you expected something else." He said, "Well what do you think I wanted?" She said, "The same thing you picked me up for the day before." He said, "I just wanted to see you. . . . If you need money I'll see you whenever you want. I'd like to see you and I'll pay you."

Moving back to her twenty-first year: After the hospitalization she took all kinds of jobs, driving a horse and buggy outside a rich Mafia restaurant on Rush Street, then working downtown at Mothers restaurant, and in the Commodity Exchange, holding the deck for two brokers in the pit: "We would sell no swine before its time," (she laughed). She worked on the options exchange. She did all sorts of things. Then she met this other guy (Man 5) whose uncle was real rich, owned a couple of blood banks and smuggled a lot of pot. Man 5 had a friend. The men were New Yorkers working in Chicago, so Boots introduced them to heroin out there and to her girlfriend. The four of them did nothing but freebase and shoot heroin. One night they were all at her girlfriend's house for dinner. Boots thought they'd been up four days. They'd gone to get some heroin, and her Man 5 fell out. They brought him back and everything was okay. Then he said he wanted to go lie down for a little while. They lay down, they sat up. Then about three, she went to wake him up, and he was in a coma. He was only twenty-four. His liver had shut down a week before. Boots recalled:

■ I remember I was working for Hammond Photography at this time. I coordinated three different magazines. I remember in the mornings, one morning in particular I looked down the hall, and Man 5 was standing in front of the toilet, but he couldn't pee. I thought something was weird, but I just lay him on the couch and gave him some cough syrup, like Vicks or something. They got him out of the coma, but after four days, he died. He was twenty-four.

Boots hastened on to the next miniplot: She was engaged to a guy in Colorado (Man 6). This boy was an angel, she recalled smiling. He was the best man at everybody's wedding. They had 180 acres in the San Juan Mountains. He ended up crashing after he was the best man at this guy's wedding. He ran off the road and broke his neck. She had gone back to Chicago. Young, wild, and not sure if she could handle a long-distance relationship, Boots had doubts about becoming a cowgirl out west. She liked the city, the fancy clothes, and if that guy were to come there (laughing), he might be out there roping down the CTA (Chicago Transit Authority) or something. She was doing some modeling at the time and she'd sent him a full-length poster of herself. Last time she went down there, his mother still hadn't touched his room, and there was Boots still hanging on the wall.

I reached for the present: "You just continued being with different guys, and at some point you started tricking?" Yes, last summer her girlfriend took her out on the street and taught her what to say and what not to say and to watch for the police.

Truth, Narrative, and Jiving

I don't know how much of Boots's story was fact and how much fiction. In the life, to jive is like to be, it's a way of talking, a way of doing. The line between fact and fiction is strategically blurred. Boots was on a fugitive's mission, and I don't think that she had any more reason to lie to me than to herself. A researcher can't ask more than that, in any situation.

Sandy is a different story, a "through no fault of her own" story. She had two hetero partners before her husband. The second one shot her in the head, saying he didn't realize the gun was loaded. Sandy is straightforward and traditional. Because Sandy fits the role of Symbolic Mother, we can imagine eventual safety for her and her kids, if not redemption. Meanwhile, Boots sweeps across the land-scape of North America, strewing dead boyfriends as she goes. She is getting closer and closer to the disposable limit:

■   About two weeks after I met her, I went to see her in Cook County Hospital. She went in for severe abdominal pain and high fever. She waited fifteen hours to be admitted. First she went to a surgical ward where they treated her well and did all kinds of tests. Then they transferred her to an internal medicine ward with cancer and AIDS patients where she had had no medical attention to speak of for the last two days. They gave her five milligrams of methadone a day for her habit; she saves these and does them all at once so she can get a little buzz. Her ex-cop friend was smuggling in street drugs to get her through, and the medical students on the surgical ward gave her new needles and alcohol. Boots wished they would give her enough methadone so that she could have used the time to kick street drugs altogether. She wants to get her life together, because by the following summer, she hopes to go wild again. She tested HIV-negative. She said.

One time in Chicago I interviewed an older woman, Ruth. She said she could write a book about her thirty years in prostitution. I later found out that she was a con, not a prostitute (she and her friend had already been interviewed by the northside station and were trying to make some money off the westside). Ruth told me some tall tales of tricks, like this girl who told her:

■ This trick picked her up one time and he was in a limousine and he told her that his boss wanted a date. She said he took her back to this mansion and drove in. She opened the door and went in. She didn't see nobody and he took her into this big room and the lights were out and she flicked on the light and there was a big casket. She said a man rose up out the casket and she screamed. When she screamed, that's when he got his kicks and he paid her and took her back. He said that was all he wanted. He would come to the neighborhood and get a new girl every time. Then all the girls got hip to him and so he had to go someplace new to get girls.

It was disconcerting not to be able to trust what people were telling me, not to be able to trust my intuition about someone with whom I had spoken at some length, like Ruth. Some people show a remarkable talent for strategic fiction. The plausibility and coherence of strategic fiction challenged my self-styled ethnographic objectivity (everything is not as simple as observing the mechanics of injection). Both observer and observed are caught in a web of partial fiction and ambiguous truths. (For example, project staff passed on the experts' simplification of the truth that HIV dies on contact with air. We also had to explain ambiguities created by HIV antibody tests that produce negative results in people who are in the early, and most infectious, stages of the disease.) The illusory and reorienting qualities of strategic fictions are in some ways similar to drug effects.

True, Ruth did *lie* about being a prostitute for thirty years. But she also had access to ethnographic data in a much more protracted sense than I, the official ethnographer. An ethnographer uses systematicity, analysis, credentials, and context to authorize her kind of truth, which is by definition based on (extended) visits. But it is only the hubris of scholars and fools that attributes more value to the truths arising out of professional visits than those of a good storyteller who has lived her life close to the scene—even if she is embellishing her character. The value of different versions of truth depends on audience and purpose.

But then again, how much is at stake in making these distinctions? Consider this little list of facts Avital Ronell (1992, 51–52) sounds out:

> Precisely because [drugs] are everywhere and can be made to do, or undo, or promise, anything. They participate in the analysis of the broken word, or a history of warfare: methedrine, or methylamphetamine, synthesized in Germany, had a determining effect inHitler's Blitzkrieg; heroin comes from *heroisch*, and Göring never went anywhere without his supply; Dr. Hubertus Strughold, father of space medicine, conducted mescaline experiments at Dachau—indeed, it would be diffi-

ESCAPE

cult to dissociate drugs from a history of modern warfare and genocide. One could begin perhaps in the contiguous neighborhood of the ethnocide of the American Indian by alcohol or strategic viral infection, and then one could never end.

There are times when it is absolutely necessary to verify as best you can the factual nature of discourse, issues of justice, for example. But in other cases it's the fictions that encode the critical truths. I can't tell you why Boots and Sandy have to fight this drug war. But I can see that it's a setup. The women fell right into the drug problem. The drug problem is *an effect* of institution, convention, and law (Ronnell 1992, 77); it preceded their particular acts. In all this, HIV is just a parasite, and whatever so-called AIDS prevention our government's got going is woefully inadequate to the task.

7 / Illusion and Control

Things don't have to get completely out of control when you are addicted. One of the first stereotypes the people on southside Chicago burst for me was this notion that when someone gets addicted to drugs they just wither in an increasingly depraved state until they roll up and die. I spoke to people in their sixties and maybe seventies who looked quite fit and who had managed decades-long heroin addictions. When the dose they needed to get high got too expensive, they'd admit themselves for a spell of treatment and reduce it. When they'd start back again, a little would go a longer way. The psychophysiological aspects of addiction, and the problems that addiction causes in one's personal and professional relationships, can to a certain extent be managed.

This chapter begins with the story of an ex-corrections officer who articulates her personal addiction management strategy, then it sinks into the (mis)management of addiction in sexual relationships, focusing on HIV risk in the lives of two women and a man. The stories come from southside Chicago field station interviews.

A Line That You Draw

In the grip of her intangible quandary, Rosalind's HIV risk seemed distant. Although she was trained as an AIDS educator when she worked in corrections, she had never faced up to the details of her own situation. She shared needles with the people with whom she started shooting, then she started using her own needles at home. Like most shooters who live with others who do not shoot, Rosalind did not bring her injection ritual to anyone's attention (she'd run a bath to cover long stays in the family bathroom). She reported having vaginal sex without condoms about once a week with three men, one of whom was Fred, the hustler who brought her to the station. He was the official sex partner in the project, because although he used heroin and karachi two to six times a week, he did not shoot it. Fred said he was having sex with, and getting money from, four other women in addition to Rosalind. He reported sex at a frequency of two to six times a week vaginally and orally without condoms. (It is revealing how discordant men's and women's memories were when it came to oral sex; men often boasted about getting it, while women claimed never having anything to do with it.) Fred might have been exposed to HIV in 1985, when he had a blood transfusion. (This was during the time when U.S. blood banks ignored mounting evidence of a yet unidentified virus poisoning the blood supply, before they began screening donors and testing blood for HIV antibodies.) Rosalind felt that the two other men with whom she had sex were safe because they didn't shoot drugs and were married. Rosalind figured they only saw their wives and her. If they were to have another woman, she would be able to tell. She would recognize the change in their behavior and schedule. Rosalind paused as she was explaining this, realizing that like many people, she did not usually think beyond the person(s) with whom she herself had sex. "Hopefully their wives are okay," she said.

What Rosalind wanted to talk about most was the career she had lost. She used to work as a corrections officer with a caseload of thirty-eight in a youth detention facility. It was she who decided who would stay, get out on parole, or be sent to maximum security; it was she who tried to keep the youth on the right path. With a Bachelor of Science degree under her belt, she thought of herself at that time of her life as ambitious and enthusiastic; firm, consistent, and fair; and definitely not scared. "The day you become scared is the day when you need to walk out the door and don't come back," she said. But things took a turn for the worse when she got hit in the mouth and an eye, when her teeth got knocked out (she didn't explain how it happened).

By the end of the Reagan era, the United States criminal justice system had reverted to its punitive foundation. Rosalind said that she was given authority but wasn't allowed to be fair. She fought to act with integrity. Pressures were insurmountable. The rougher she and her coworkers were with the youths, the more the administration viewed them as being on top of their job. But she always insisted on a good reason for sending someone to solitary; she never used anybody as a scapegoat. She scooped up all her fury and held it inside. Sometimes she felt like "damn, I just got to have something going to deal with this. I can't deal with this and think being sober." She escaped into heroin, breathing in the sensory pleasures of illusory release.

Rosalind lived a double life in addictions and corrections: "You get high or whatever and hang out. And then you come home and you go to bed. You take a bath. You get up in the morning. You put your clean clothes on. You get your briefcase and go to your job and play that role." Heroin was an upper for her. Nobody at work ever knew she was high. She'd walk around and they'd say, "Gee, you're in a great mood today!" When she took heroin, she was ready to go, and that's why she got into it. But she felt her superior started to single her out for minor infractions like being a few minutes late. Rosalind realized that her superiors got to stay in their jobs by disparaging the folks over whom they had authority. She resigned before they had time to build a case against her and felt that she beat them at their own game. At least she knew that she could not withstand scrutiny. This way, she could still go back anytime she got ready.

Four years had passed since the corrections job, by the time I talked to her. She was still angry at herself: "If I had of played my cards right and hadn't got involved in bullshit, I would have been a whole lot further. . . . I got to think about now, how I have to get control over this." Rosalind used drugs steadily by then (Fred said that it was hard for her to get motivated without them). She was also a strong and pragmatic woman and knew the value of self-discipline. She had started injecting drugs about six months before the interview with people she met through her outpatient substance abuse program. She was at their house and someone came in and had some cocaine and they were doing it. Rosalind asked if she could snort some, but they said they didn't have enough for snorting. So it was either not getting high or doing it the way they were doing it. She shared their needles.

The high felt the same as when she snorted (tooted) it. She felt bad about shooting the first time, knew it would magnify her problem. Rosalind told herself that she wouldn't do it anymore. But then she wanted to see if she could get the feeling that they said they got. Since it wasn't any great feeling the first time, she tried it again. She really didn't get the feeling the second time, so she tried it again and found it a little bit better. That's how the injecting began. (Goaded on into the mist by the pleasure cries of acquaintances, the drugs illusionary powers blossom even as they bind their molecular structure to your cells and to your soul.)

The method of administration—whether smoking, tooting, or shooting may not change the quality of the high so much as the velocity of onset, duration, side effects, and cost. Different people have different responses to the same drug; response can be manipulated according to method of administration. In other words, choosing a method of administration isn't necessarily about getting a better high. Rosalind explains:

■   See, when you take cocaine it's just about the rush, all right? Shooting cocaine intravenously I'm able to control it better so far as not going off, okay? If I was to smoke cocaine, freebase cocaine, if I had seven hundred dollars, I'd smoke seven hundred dollars. But if I were to take cocaine intravenously, I would maybe spend about eighty dollars or something like that, and that would be it and I wouldn't be all paranoid. I wouldn't be all hyped up or anything like that, like dealing. And I could go and sit down and be mellow. Whereas if I had smoked cocaine, I'd have adverse reactions such as being extremely hyper. Very active. My eyes are popped. Paranoid.

Rosalind wasn't making up examples. She learned a sobering lesson the time she blew seven hundred dollars and worked hard to control her addiction without exceeding her resources:

■   I never broke into nobody's store and took anything. I never stole from my parents. I never took furniture and TVs. I have a house full of furniture. Living room, dining room, bedroom, bathroom, kitchen. I have the best of stuff. I have Sony stereo systems, Sansui speakers, floor model TV, Zenith remote control. VCR, double head. I never take my stuff out the house and sell it. Someplace you have to have a line that you draw. And when you've gotten up to that line, then it's no more that you can do and even if you do want it. And I've wanted it, too. But you just have to, there's no more money, there's nothing else you can do. It's over. Take your ass to bed.

[Doesn't the dope compel you to do things that you really don't want to do? There are contradictory feelings, right?] It does, it has, it compels me to do a lot of things, but I don't do them. I know how far I'm gon' go, like anybody that smokes cocaine. If I had seven hundred dollars, I'd smoke up the whole seven hundred dollars. I have smoked up my whole paycheck and walked out of there with fifty cents and had to pay my bills. I had to go to my savings account and take seven hundred dollars out of my savings account and put it back in my checking account. [And how long did it take to smoke seven hundred dollars?] A day, a night. [And what did it feel like?] You feel like a piece of

shit. [What do you feel like when you're doing it?] You just want another hit. . . . But I didn't go into my house and get my stereo or my
television or nothing. The money was gone. That's it. It's over with. I've
already fucked up enough. I spent my whole check. Now I got to replace that money to pay my bills. I even had a guy tell me he would
give me some cocaine if he held my car keys until I bring his money
back. Or whenever I pay him, he'll give me my car. I told him, I say,
"Man, I don't want no cocaine that bad. It's not worth that. Naw. You
can't hold my car." . . . I had a brand new red . . . [sportscar].

Rosalind was living at her mother's house when we spoke, along
with a sister and nephew. She was resentful that since she had become
an addict and given up her job, she had become the family scapegoat.
Her father, a white-collar supervisor, used to be an alcoholic; when
she was a child, she was embarrassed by the other children's jokes
about his intoxicated state. Since the doctor told him he would kill
himself if he didn't stop drinking with his diabetes, he quit. But
Rosalind said that that sure didn't mean he dealt with the underlying
emotional problems any better than she. He was a dry drunk, unre-
solved feelings ready to put him in the same old boat anytime something traumatic happened. She felt that her parents exacerbated her
obsessive-compulsive behaviors; that if she had had cancer, they
could have seen what she had as an illness and learn how to help her.
But because her illness seized on dope, they constantly criticized her,
feeding a vicious cycle:

■   Their concept is, in which they're so wrong, is that "it's not my
problem; it's your problem." But it's all of our problems, because my
pain has ran over into their cup. So they have certain pains and wounds
too that need to be healed. So it's just like we get to arguing and we
both go at each other and say things and no one hears the other.
You're just throwing out the hurt but you're never trying to heal it.

Rosalind received income from disability as well as from two men friends. Fred, whom I had interviewed first, said that Rosalind worked the street sometimes. He said that she had "certain tricks that she will go and see . . . she is not a straight out stomp down prostitute, but she has her friends that she calls." Nonetheless, she was offended when I referred to her men friends as "tricks" early in my interview with her. Later I apologized and asked her to explain how the money thing worked in her sexual friendships:

■ They give me money. So I don't really think that you have a clear picture of what's going on. . . . I think that you think that I have sex with them and they just give me money. They say "here." And that's it, right? These individuals I've known for years and years. I used to go with them, okay? So we know each other very well. Our relationship is not strictly a sexual thing. We do other things. And a lot of times, I have sex with them and they don't give me any money, okay? I may say, "Well, Jake, I would like to get my clothes out of the cleaners," and he'll say, "Okay. Fine. I'll get them out." Or I need to get my stereo out the shop. He'll get it out. Like that. It's not like we have sex, and then he says, "Here's twenty dollars" and that's it, you know.

Her situation demonstrates one of the keys to a nuanced definition of prostitution. Whether or not the label of prostitute is appropriate depends on the extent to which social interaction shrinks around the sex act. Professional sex acts are more focused on a ritual of exchange, a coordinated sequence of acts so well known that even strangers who do not share the same spoken language are fluent in the language of sex for hire: solicitation, negotiation (of act-money-condom use), monetary exchange, sex (and possibly body fluid exchange), return, and separation. In contrast, nonprofessional sex acts tend to be more embedded in social life. Sexual scripts are there, but they are more complex, assume more variation with person and place, and take more time to develop. A more accurate way of classifying particular women as prostitutes would consider the degree of focus on the sex act itself.[1]

Rosalind was tired of being an addict; she wanted a job, to start earning money, complete her master's degree, and move on with her life. But she had lost her drive. She didn't care about the nice house and clothes, the charge accounts for Marshall Fields, Lord and Taylor, and Carson's that used to matter so much. She wasn't ready:

■   In order to have a job, you have to have yourself together. You can't go in there half stepping. You can't go in there with your hands swollen. You can't go in their with marks all over. And you have to be looking presentable. And you have to be able to function. . . . I'm trying to get ready. I'm trying my damndest to get ready. This has really, really, really fucked my life up.

Rosalind was afraid that any money she earned she'd blow on dope. She felt safer not making any. If she put herself to the test, she might have sunk deeper. So she held on to her measure of self-control—keeping her material goods and not boosting anyone else's—copped her stuff, and ranted at this future on hold. Rosalind had met the harsh judgment of the state head on and was both favored and punished. Enslaved by the magic powders, she could no longer perform as agent of state. She slipped into the wrong side of the mirror and lost her alibi. (People in power don't run out of alibis.) The thing is, no matter which side of the game you're on—officer or addict—you're still only a pawn in the power game.

Networking

HIV infection hit the injecting drug-using networks in Chicago before people knew much of anything about the virus. Nat was one of the regulars at the southside station and had heard all the standard warnings. He distrusted government information, not believing that it was safe to shake hands or touch someone with AIDS, to eat in a restaurant where the cook has AIDS, or to use public toilets. But given the extent to which injectors recognized dirty needles as a threat by 1988, chances were Nat wouldn't reuse someone else's needle without cleaning it with bleach first, or hand someone his used needle without cleaning or comment.[2] I do not know if he was HIV-positive or not; he did say he was at high risk for AIDS. He also said he never thinks of using condoms; he felt that he had no reason to as his sex partner was not promiscuous. (He must have been referring to the elder of the two sex partners he brought in to be interviewed at the station [Maggie]; for the statement did not describe the younger [Simone].) The discrepant levels of awareness regarding the risk of dirty needles compared to the risk of sex without condoms reflects a number of factors, including the fact that gay men and injectors were the first to be hit in the United States, as well as the relative ease of changing drug-use behavior compared to sexual behavior. I didn't get Nat's story—he kept nodding off during the interview, so I had to cut it off. But through interviews with Maggie and Simone, it became clear how his sexual activities linked the fates of these two women.

Step by Step
Until she watched her nephew suffer and die, Maggie didn't know much about AIDS. She went to Cook County hospital every day. At first she was afraid to kiss him, though she did anyway so he wouldn't feel bad. She stopped being concerned about getting infected herself after the nurses answered all her questions. Her nephew was gay, and the family took that as a hard blow. So was her baby brother. She couldn't really accept it, although she knew it was his life. Her brother chose it, and she loved him. When her sister's son got AIDS, that upset the family. She had another sister with a gay daughter, and that was doing a job on them too. That sister started drinking, then later got herself together again. This is what happened to Maggie's nephew:

■   Right. Well, when we first found out that he had AIDS, we didn't believe it because maybe you know something is there and you don't really want to believe it. And when he told us he had suffered with this cough for so long, but we still kept saying it was pneumonia, pneumonia. Just a cold, you know. He'll get over this cold. He'll get over this cold. And it was getting worser, and he was losing so much weight. And he didn't . . . they say some AIDS patients suffers with it a long time but, you know, when he told us that he had it, actually he suffered maybe three months, and then, but I didn't want to believe it. We knew it was there. We often thought about it. I even mentioned it to his sisters. Then we'd say, after all, it's just a cold, he'll get over it once they get him in the hospital, give him some strong medications. He'll get over it. Finally, it took him a long time to even admit that he had it, too. It took him actually three weeks before his death that he admitted it. Because, first my nieces told me doctors said it was cancer. So, we thought it was cancer, at first, and then after they, I guess, quieted it down a little bit, they let him come home and we had to rush him back to the hospital maybe about a couple weeks after he had came home. And he, when I went to see him, he cried and hugged me and he told me to forgive him for what he has made of his life. And I had told him that it wasn't for me to forgive him, it was up to God to forgive him. And I told him to just ask God to forgive him for what he had made of his life, for what he's done to himself. So, he just, you know, after he saw what was really going on in his life, and I guess he might have really knew it but he just didn't want to accept it. But, like I said, in the three weeks before he passed, he told us all that he had AIDS. And we were very upset. We were all upset cause we had just lost my mom, and here he was on his deathbed. It's too much to watch him suffer the way AIDS ate up his body. I don't know how to really tell you. He never was no size, but I guess when he passed, he weighed maybe seventy-eight pounds. . . . You could see every bone in his body, every bone in his body. He went into a coma, but he was strong, and I guess because we were there for him, it was always somebody there. They let us come to the hospital whenever we wanted to and we could stay as long as we wanted. My sister spent the night with him and she's a nurse, so she took care of her own child. He went into a coma and he stayed that way for about four days and he came back and he could talk a little bit and he'd slurp a little bit, but he knew us. He knew who we were. The doctors told us that part of his brain had died. And when I would touch his forehead, he would be hot everywhere but up around that area 'cause they say part of his brain had died there. And it was just where he couldn't walk no more, he couldn't eat no more.

Oh, the nurses were nice and supportive. . . . He had one doctor, I can't remember her name. She was a woman, and she was so sweet. She explained to us things that a two-year-old knew what she was talking about. She explained it to us step by step what was going to happen. And everything happened just like she said. . . . One while, sometimes, in the room would be maybe almost fifteen people and they wouldn't complain. They put him in a private room. They wouldn't say anything when we all would come to see him. It would get so after he did come out of that coma, though, he wouldn't talk too much because he said he would get tired. So, we wouldn't let him talk. We'd just come and he would stare at us. And the ones that he really knew very well, and I was one of his favorite aunts, he'd didn't never want us to leave. He'd get mad, though. You could see that frown on his face, you know, and I'd tell him "I've got to go, I'm tired." I gotta come from work and I done stayed till eleven or twelve o'clock at the hospital, and I'm tired. I'm doing this everyday, you know. But he would say okay. But by his mother spending the night, he would finally accept us leaving, but knowing she would be there with him. Then his last request, he wrote a beautiful letter to the family. The nurse wrote it for him. He had requested could he go home and the doctors didn't want him to go 'cause they knew he was dying. He kept saying he wanted to go home, wanted to go home. So she let him come. So, we brought him home. He stayed one day and that night we had to rush him back to the hospital. And when we rushed him back, the next day he had passed. But we felt good because he did come home. And then he would say . . . who knows what when you die what you see. 'Cause he told us the day before he died that my mother and my father, they're both deceased, were waiting for him and he was ready to go to Grandmama and Daddy and he passed on. But the blessing part of it [crying] . . . that's part of it. The blessing part of it is he's not suffering and, we knowed he really suffered. We know that. And, like I say, that is the blessed part of it. He's not suffering and now he's at rest. I just pray now that I hope my brother, you know, by him being gay, doesn't catch AIDS. All I can do is hope. He had a friend who had AIDS. Now, that's why I'm afraid. Because his friend died of AIDS.

Maggie lost her nephew, her mother, and a first cousin that year. She had already given up on her relationship with Nat before he brought her into the southside station for an interview. When her mother lay dying, he had disappeared, and that was the last straw. She couldn't stand when he taunted her for being out with other men, which she wasn't, or spending time with all the sissies, the gay men she sang with in the church choir. She wanted him out of her apartment. The empty cartons were sitting in the hallway waiting for him to pack.

When injectors first meet potential lovers, their habit of drug administration is not usually part of their presentation of self (unless they meet through a dealer or other injectors). Non-injecting partners do find out eventually; how long it takes depends on how hip they are and how badly they want to know. If non-injecting partners are already into snorting or smoking dope, they might start shooting too. Some break the relationship off as soon as they find out. If they care about the person and want to stay together, but don't want to shoot drugs themselves, a compromise is found. One way to reduce conflict is for the shooter to always carry out injection-related activities elsewhere. Out of sight, out of mind, makes for steady relationships. Unfortunately, this compromise tends to inhibit conversations about injecting, HIV risk, and condoms. I believe it was like that between Maggie and Nat before she got fed up. One thing about Nat though, he was one of the few injectors who was willing to bring his sex partners in to the station to be interviewed and tested. Most of the others didn't want to deal with their partners' questions about risk. Not only did the interviews provoke a conversation about the sore subject of injecting; now there was a lethal virus messing with the balance in their relationships.

Maggie first met Nat where she worked at the medical center. She didn't find out he shot dope until almost a year of dating. She wasn't looking to find out, and he seemed all right. She would spend the night at his house, and he would go out, come back; they'd talk and laugh. He would say he was going to take care of some business for the landlord or get something to eat, and then he'd stay out two, three hours. He did tell her that he was going to a methadone program not long after they started dating. So she knew he used to be addicted but figured the methadone was taking care of him.

■ It was about two years after [we met], he had some Valium on him and the police picked him up and the bottle was in his sister's name. So, he was put in jail and during that time, they were tearing down the building that he was living in and I didn't want his furniture and clothes to be thrown out in the streets and that's how he got with me. I brought him to my house. He stayed in jail for about a month because his sister was very ill. We had to get her to sign the papers, get it notarized, get the doctor to sign the papers, get it notarized, get all this done, but anyway, finally they let him out. The reason they had raised his bond so high because he was an addict and of his past record and that's why it was too high to get him out. I would run to try to deal with these papers for him and I knew he didn't do anything because that's what they had him in there for. They let him out and he came straight to my house and that's how he got in my house because I really didn't want him to come live with me, see, because of his background. My children didn't really know nothing about drugs, in that sense. I'm not saying they don't know nothing about it 'cause some of them are grown, but it never was brought in my house. Not even cigarettes. Not even my children smoke. When he came, he was so nice to them, he was very nice to them and he never done anything in my home. . . .

But one day he came in from out in the streets and he was just different. Just different. I guess maybe I set down and really looked at him. I confronted him about it and then he finally told me the truth. He said, "I do it every once in a while." I said, "Okay, but I don't want it in my house" because we don't do this here. Drugs don't come up in this house. So we didn't do it. He would respect me in that sense and he wouldn't do it in the house.

Maggie was the law in her house. Her rules barring drug use served to protect her and her children from the threatening sadness of addiction. It would not protect her from AIDS, however. She had been having sex with Nat about once a week until seven months before the interview, when she decided she didn't want to be bothered with him anymore. She had never used a condom in her life. At forty-six, she'd had three kids, a tubal ligation, and until she saw her nephew die, nary a thought about the relevance of AIDS in her own life. She had no reason to think this gay men's disease may have been in her bed: In 1989, the idea that women could become HIV-infected was not actively clear in the minds of many North Americans, despite the one-male-to-one-female ratio of infection in Africa and the Caribbean. But Nat may have put her at risk of HIV. He may have used an infected needle at some point, or he may have gotten infected from Simone, the other twenty-three-year-old sex partner he brought in to the southside station.

Home from College for the Summer
I'd learned in the surveillance interview with Simone that in the last six months she'd had three boyfriends and ten tricks, including eight regulars with whom she'd had vaginal and oral sex. She used con-

doms only with tricks, only for vaginal, and not oral, sex; she never used condoms with personal partners, not even with Nat, whom she knew was an injector. We explored the history and present context of these facts in the ethnographic interview that followed.

Simone entered the land of risk when she was sixteen and raped. She said the first time she heard about AIDS, she wondered if she caught it then, if the virus was out back in 1980. The rapist was Belizean or Jamaican, she said that she couldn't pin down the accent. She was at a party with her girlfriends. The eldest was eighteen and supposed to chaperone. So the girls left the Cabrini-Green housing projects where Simone lived and went up north. They were hanging out with a group of Belizeans or Jamaicans, getting high and talking. She was sitting on the porch waiting for her girlfriends, because they knew the area well and she was a newcomer. She didn't really know the guys she'd met. It started getting dark. Her girlfriends had all gone somewhere, to the store. It had really gotten dark. It was around the same time of year as the interview, December, and dark came fast. She was sitting there, and all of a sudden somebody put their hands over her mouth and eyes and pulled her in the hallway and it happened. She said it went on for about an hour, with her screaming and hollering and nobody helping her. She still had nightmares about it.

Simone said she'd been raped before, earlier, when she was about eight, by her father. She told her mother. In a rage, her mother told Simone she must have liked it. That really hurt her. She distanced herself from her family. By twelve she turned to liking sex for money and started learning about the street. She specialized in older men like Nat (who was sixty-two at the time), with whom she felt safe. Until she met Nat, her relationships with guys had never worked out. All through her teens, she was turned off by sex and felt depressed and ignorant. She started using alcohol and marijuana. She went out with a cocaine baser for a while and tried the pipe. She knew she was doing it to belong, and it made her vomit. By nineteen or twenty she

111

started using Sherman Stick (PCP, or angel dust). She didn't like hallucinogens because they made her feel totally outside her character; the day after tripping, she wouldn't know what she'd done. So then she tried heroin, karachi, snorting it, every day, every day. This kept her in an animated state. She explained about karachi, how it had been around Chicago

■   . . . a good probably five years, but nobody really started using it up until about two years ago. Because it was like they would use blow, which is another form of heroin. It's [karachi] the snorter's form, instead of the shooter's form. They went from blow and added more barbiturates to it and made it into karachi. It is habit forming, very. A lot of people don't know that they are addicted to it until like, maybe you could go for a day and you would think maybe the reason why your stomach is cramping or your back is hurting or you got a cold chill is because you're coming down with a flu or a cold, but, it's really withdrawal symptoms from the drugs.

In contrast to Simone, Rosalind, the former corrections officer, hated karachi. She said it was made of pills, barbiturates, and if she wanted to take some pills, she wouldn't have someone mash them up for her to snort up. But it was quite popular at that time in Chicago. Simone got into heroin with her brother:

■   We've always been like two and two, whatever he do, I do. He was using and he start selling it, just like the coke. He was using the coke, snorting it, just like he was selling it. I got off into the business with him. We had quite a few business dealings over the summer. . . . Every summer when he would come home from college and I would come home from college and we would get high all summer. So one summer, which was the summer of last year, I snorted a gross of twelve bags by myself. I had acquired a habit of six bags a day within a thirty-day period. I started snorting more and more every day. Until

one day I was sitting down and I was snorting, and this particular day
I snorted about twelve bags the night before. The next day I snorted
about eight bags by myself. This is not with somebody else, this is by
myself. As I was in the bathroom doing my hair, I was curling my hair.
All of a sudden blood just shot out of my nose and I found it had ate
away a lot of tissue in my nose. It's just healing up now. My nose is
swollen up like a tomato. [So you stopped after that?] So I stopped.
As I stopped I had withdrawal symptoms. . . . vomiting, massive bowel
movements like diarrhea, but it was solid, it wasn't liquid form. It was
like . . . I was real dazed. I couldn't stand on my own two feet for
maybe like three days. Then after seventy-two hours it just gradually
went away. Within five days that habit was kicked without no Met
[methadone] or nothing. It was like cold turkey, kicked it by myself.

I stayed in the house for maybe a week and my skin started to
clear back up. . . . I did it all by myself, all by myself. That made me
know that I was much more stronger than I gave myself credit for. I
realized that a lot of young people come in contact with these drugs
and the most times they get high, it's because it's free. And by it being
free doesn't mean it's good for you. [Well it's free for a little while. . . .]
Yeah, for just a little while. Then you might start having . . . that's another reason why I was turning tricks to support my habit. [How did
that come about? One day you just decided, I need some money, I'm
going to turn a trick?] Okay. Like one of my professors at school liked
me and I had developed this habit. He would like, I know a lot of girls
that was going to school with me were turning dates with a lot of the
professors? [For money or grades?] Money and grades. Because a lot of
them, their parents weren't too well off and maybe the only reason
why they were at this university was because of a scholarship . . . and
the little jobs that they had off campus wasn't paying that much. One
of my roommates told me she knew a way I could get a quick three
hundred dollars. The less fee I ever charged for a date is fifteen dollars.
And the highest I ever got was three hundred dollars. This three hundred dollars would come like every other two days from different

people. I was doing pretty good. I had a habit of something like five bags [of karachi] a day, which was a hundred dollars a day.

[You got that in rural Illinois?] No, my brother would bring it to me. Like on the weekends he would bring me something like, I'd say, a good thirty-five bags. That is how I was paying for it. I was selling the other and I used myself. What he didn't know is that I developed such a habit that when he found out, it was too late.

Simone's brother was buying his drugs from another ambiguously identified Belizean or Jamaican man. She said that both she and her brother stopped using it, that she might smoke a joint every once in a while. (She must have forgotten that she'd already told me during the surveillance interview that she had slipped back into chipping.) Simone felt that she could whittle her way through a lot, even out there with the whores who turn dates for two dollars. She used her education like a shield: "Now you cannot take a prostitute and make her a housewife, just like you can't take a whore and make her a college grad." Most of her partners are regulars, older men who may have business, dope dealers.

After the ethnographic interview moved through the round of guy and drug stories (including one about an occasional sex partner who was mostly living in Germany with a pregnant wife), Simone returned to her early rape experience:

■ So it was like the man was too oversize for my body. I had never really had sex before. I was so sore for so long. It's like when I first went to the hospital I had like seventeen stitches from the front and seventeen stitches backward. I had ten stitches in my behind. [Did they ever catch this guy?] No, never did. And to make it so bad he brought me all the way to my house and I was up north, and he took me all the way to my house. I wanted to know why did he want to know where I lived at so bad. [So you were scared he would come back.] Yeah, I wouldn't go out for a long time, by myself or with nobody else.

I started my freshman year, my sophomore year, at age seventeen be-cause I wouldn't go back outside. I just wouldn't. I didn't want no men around me period, not even my brothers. I didn't trust them either, because what had happened to me in my earlier years and I still was kind of against men before then, but I handled it, without a psychiatrist. Because like after I got raped they had to take me to the hospital, be-cause like all the time while I was in this man's cab . . . I can remember that he had a cab, and all the time while I was in this cab I was bleeding real heavy. I had on like a white pair of pants like a snow suit. My whole pair of pants was full of blood. . . . He had hit me in my face and loos-ened my teeth so I couldn't scream no more. My face was real bruised. When I got halfway to where I live at, he push me out of the cab. I managed to walk home. A lot of people say that they don't know how I made it that far the way I was bleeding. I lost maybe, two pints of blood. The policeman that handled my case and the detective, they say they are still pursuing him. I still keep in close contact with them. I got to see his face. I will never forget it. I will know right now to this day, if I ever see him again. They say I was lucky that he didn't kill me. . . . He left me there to bleed to death, because he knew that I was bleeding like that. I know it was all over him. I scratched him in his face. My nails were twice as long as they are now. I had flesh caked under my nails. I know that I disfigured his face and his neck and his stomach. I mean he actually took all his clothes off. He really, really enjoyed that. It's like whoever his wife or the one that he's with now, he beats them, be-cause he really enjoyed that. If I ever see him again, I will kill him. That would be my justice. I hate to say that, because I don't want to take anybody's life.

Conditions at the Front

In Chicago, it was commonly thought that if you are addicted to snorting heroin and you are around people who shoot, unless you have needle phobia, you'll probably start shooting too. Efficient and cost-effective, the initial switch temporarily eases hustling responsi-bilities. If you are a shooter, as Rosalind had recently become, you need to be part of a social network of other shooters with whom you share information about copping sites and drug quality (tooters tended to have distinct but overlapping networks). Shooters in the same social network may also share drugs, a place to shoot, bleach, water, cotton, and works—and in this variety of contexts and me-dia—HIV. By hooking up with a network of souls who shoot, you also hook up with a network of bodies who are susceptible to becom-ing infected via repeated injections of drug-blood solutions of HIV. (There is almost always a residue of blood left over in a uncleaned used needle, whether it carries heroin or penicillin or polio vaccine.) [3]

As an epidemiological category in the NIDA-sponsored AIDS dem-onstration project, the conception of sex partner that I was given to work with grew out of a concern that women were underrepresented in outreach efforts. Official concern was part of a larger effort to in-crease awareness of women's HIV risk, but the category of sex partner was weakened by a stereotypical notion that sex partners were female innocent victims of licentious male injectors.[4] As it turned out, how-ever, the largest sample of sex partners whom I was able to recruit were neither especially innocent nor female. Half of the sex partners I interviewed were men who had sex with women who injected (such as Rosalind's partner Fred). Almost half of the sex partners were ha-bitual users of heroin and/or cocaine in tooted or smoked form; about one out of three were addicted to heroin, mostly in karachi form (like Simone). In contrast, one out of five sex partners were abstinent, spurning both drugs and alcohol (like Maggie).

The pattern of HIV risk is complicated by both the diversity of involvements in the drug scene and the sexual cross-links. Both these dimensions of risk change historically. So, for example, by the begin-ning of the nineties, crack had transformed the demographics and epidemiology of HIV risk on the southside.[5] The social networks of mostly older heads who injected heroin, which dominated the Forty-

Seventh Street market in the late 1980s, gave way to a more youth-dominated drug market. The pharmacology altered the pattern of sexual risk as well, from heroin's mellow suppression of libido to cocaine's manic excesses.

Because Simone tooted rather than shot drugs, she was not directly at risk of HIV as a result of drug administration (aside from the fact that addiction generally suppresses immune system response). If there was HIV circulating in the southside shooting networks, she may have indirectly exposed herself by having unprotected vaginal sex with Nat. In contrast to Simone, who did not shoot dope but was nevertheless active in the drug subculture, Maggie was a square, respectable single mother who liked to sing in the church choir and who never got high at all, not even on alcohol. Maggie had also put herself at risk of HIV infection by having unprotected vaginal intercourse with Nat. And via Nat, she was also susceptible to the paths of exposure opened up by Simone and her clients and boyfriends (see fig. 1).

The conditions created by the drug-war market affected patterns of social organization and patterns of HIV risk. Keeping injection equipment illegal directly increased the probability that people would reuse needles and hence that HIV would circulate among shooters and their sexual partners. In addition, the illegality of heroin and cocaine dependency has wider, more complex effects. In low-income neighborhoods where the drug market stands in for more useful and healthy economic formations, no one is free from the consequences of addiction. Rosalind, Fred, Maggie, Nat, and Simone all had non-addicted family and friends on whom they relied for emotional and material support. The imagery of deviance and unlawfulness multiplies their problems, compounding the stresses of interpersonal relationships and aggravating (even as they arise from) social divisions between those in the drug subculture and those in the mainstream. The criminalization of addiction physically separates drug users by incarcerating them; our jails and prisons are overflowing with them.

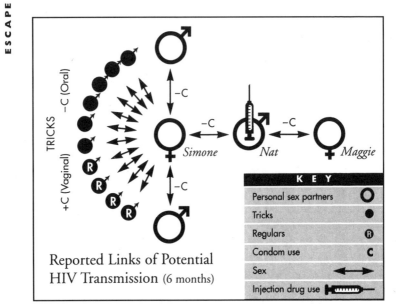

Reported Links of Potential
HIV Transmission (6 months)

Figure 1. Diagram showing exported links of potential HIV.

In the free world, criminalization induces strategies of impression management that tend to hamper communication and increase HIV risk in the most intimate relationships.

As the drug war raged, AIDS had a running start right through the heart of the nation. At twenty-three, Simone worked the streets carrying the knowledge of her brief time at college like a good luck charm (drug- and sex-filled though it was). At thirty-eight, Rosalind yearned for a life of stability and order, but couldn't go back to work bearing the stigmata of addiction. At forty-six, Maggie walled herself off with church and family, even as she watched her gay nephew die. Biochemicals, sexual intimacy, and religious song: Each woman found some solace as she beat back the pain and dealt with the risks.

8 / Easter in Livingston

> *This is the state of simulation, a state in which we are obliged
> to replay all scenarios precisely because they have all taken
> place already, whether actually or potentially. . . . We live in
> an interminable reproduction of ideals, phantasies, images and
> dreams which are now behind us, yet which we must continue
> to reproduce in a sort of inescapable indifference.*
> —*Jean Baudrillard,* After the Orgy

On the evening of Good Friday, we walked the long hill down to town, trying to find the man who fixes motors, ours having cut out part way across the bay between Punta Gorda, Belize, and Livingston, Guatemala. The side street was lined with homes and businesses, few if any people or cars. Cipher and I had arrived the day before. He was a Garifuna Rasta man from around there and knew many people. We were still a ways from town when we saw a woman, a man, no, a woman, sitting on the stone wall near the grocery. She saw Cipher and approached, enveloping us in her tall frame, her skinny arms lounging on our shoulders. Her voice was low and rough, her face manly, but she gestured sex like a woman. Her skimpy blouse and skirt were old and unclean. My eyes wandered to her throat, searching for the indisputable Adam's apple.

This search for the Adam's apple seems important somehow, illustrating an impulse for categorization, something about my need to fit something—like a body—into the concept of man or woman or man-woman before I could relax and listen to what anyone was saying. The impulse for categorization is useful—it underlies our ability to be systematic, and hence to do science and law. But sometimes it gets in the way, or leads down paths that may be more easily thinkable but not necessarily germane. Like the drug war representations of marijuana, crack, and heroin as all equally evil, while alcohol and prescription drug addiction is unfortunate, but okay. Or the categorization of AIDS as a gay, Haitian, or sexual disease: partial truths that can sometimes be more misleading than lies. So I was running a loose life experiment, attempting to suspend my impulse to categorize. On this day, I decided to ignore the Adam's apple and embrace the contradictions of culture and biology. But over the next few days I did jot down occasional notes about people and events, always after the fact, in private.

The transvestite attractions of Easter in Livingston were well known in certain parts of the world. Earlier that year, when I was interviewing people in Punta Gorda about AIDS, I spoke to a young Garifuna woman who had visited family in Livingston the year before. This is what she told me:

■   There's a lot of [Garifuna] guys in Livingston that dress up like woman. I saw them. Anytime I go. The year before I went there and I saw a lot of them there. They dress up like woman, all their shoes, their fingernails. They have long fingernails. Their hair, they fix it like woman. Lipstick, everything. The only way you can find out it's a man is from the muscles on their foot. You can see the difference. . . . They don't like to come to PG because people in PG tease them. They make fun of them. And they find guys there, some of them white people. I think they come from United States, and from Guatemala City too. But there are lots of them that find these guys that are homo-

sexual. They go with them. You see them going with them holding
hands on the side of the sea beach. I saw them a lot.

Easter there will be a lot of people there. On Easter time lots of
people go from here to there. Because on that time they crucify Jesus,
they do the act. . . . they crucify Jesus and [perform] the way of the
cross. All of that they do. From the night it starts when you are looking
for Jesus . . . the following morning that's when they start, when he's
backing the cross on his back, and they have, just the way they say it in
the Bible, they have some guys that are standing beside him, watching
him. And they put the prickle on his head. And they put like stains, like
blood is dripping off, they start to whip him, they whip him and they do
it through the street and it hot, hot, hot, hot, hot. And some people
are crying, and the night after Jesus have already died when they put
him in the tomb, they walk with the coffin and the statue, they walk
him through the streets. They go to Church and all. It's good. And then
they have a dance after that. Big thing. Good. Livingston. It's not far
from here. Usually the boat leaves here at three and it reaches Livingston about 5:30.

You'd think things would be calmer in the tropics—palm trees
swaying in the sunset beach breeze, lounge chair, long legs, and
drinks like the ads that train North American vacation desires. Livingston might have been an out-of-the-way place, but it was lively
and not particularly peaceful, not normally. At least it wouldn't be
billed in the United States as a nice Disneyfied family spot. And this
was Easter, time of transformation, death, resurrection, and wild partying. The diverse mix of Garifuna, Kekchi Maya, and Spanish
townspeople were joined by Garifuna who came up the coast from
Honduras and across the bay from Belize in dories and public ferries;
Kekchi Maya who walked and canoed downriver from mountain villages; Spanish men and their families from Guatemala City who arrived in pleasure boats; light-skinned tourists with backpacks from
Europe and the states who came by jet through some regional capital

in a nostalgic search for reality in the primitive. (There are no roads to Livingston.)

By the time we arrived in the center of town, the man-Christ bearing the cross had already been whipped down the street. Scary. Why do people reenact this famous act of immolation? And by whose logic is it accompanied by multitudinous, multiracial sexual acts? I understood the Christ story in Central America as an overlay, incorporated into ceremonies of transformation born centuries before, here between the Mayans' mountain spirits and the lost lands of Africa. Fused in the violence of conquest, these ancestral presences retained distinct cultural preferences; the unique character of the Central American carnivalesque grew from millions of details, ranging from matters of address to the intimacies of sex.

The crowd was not so much an audience in an outdoor Christian theater as a source of energy pulling deep from history and spirit. There seemed to be a great hummmmmmm, a buzz hovering over the moving mass. Bystanders watched, mingling with the core procession bearing larger-than-life icons of death and religiosity. Every few yards, a Lion tried to attack the dead statue of Christ as it lay flat in a glass coffin. Framed in wood, decorated with greens and hibiscus, you could see its white shrouded body and beard inside, a needle floating through the multitudes. Behind it came the giant Mary and the saints, their long black robes matching the black dresses of the old women in the crowd below.

Biblical actors mime an imaginative history, but the behind-the-scene orgasms must have been real enough. Observing the procession gave me an embodied sense of what demographers and epidemiologists refer to as "population." The potential for the intermingling of body fluids in a crowd this size was mind-boggling. I was trying to comprehend the enormity of the still-latent epidemic and worried about the implications of boisterous partying that enveloped the ritual icons.

The cantinas were full. Everybody was out promenading, sitting along the curbs talking, laughing, drinking, eating, fighting, smoking, dancing, wheeling and dealing. The old Spanish whores were in the Sweet River Bar servicing the foreign seamen off the shrimp boats. We went to Cipher's aunt's house to see his cousin the tailor, who was ailing. They say his illness was caused by professional jealousy; someone allegedly poisoned him because they wanted his business. Cipher began his cure and prescribed herbs. The middle-aged man looked bloated and sickly. (He was buried about a month after Easter.) We ate some cooked shrimp and joined the street action again, running into an uncle who wanted a drink although he was already quite drunk and so we went inside another cantina. Later we drank with some other men in a pizza place where there was some question as to whether men at a neighboring table were government spies. And so went the night, bar to bar to bar.

The next day, Saturday of Glory, we reentered the party scene on the ocean beach. Local Garifuna boys dressed up in tight, bright sexy clothes were milling about middle-aged Guatemalan gentlemen in fine shirts and gold jewelry, some aggressive, some furtive. The man-to-man scene was taking place right in the midst of hot hetero interactions. The action filled up all the little tables lined up on the sand in the shade of the thatch-roofed cantinas, spilling out toward the ocean, complementing the soka and salsa music blaring from the speakers. If they were there, the transvestites blended into the scene.

Later, we sat at a little stand that serves fish dinners up the street from the dock, where the ferry boat comes in from Puerto Barrios, across from the big luxury hotel. (At this point in time, Puerto Barrios already had the distinction of being the site of the largest seizure of cocaine in Central American history, i.e., 2,400 kilograms in 1987 [Scott and Marshall 1991, 187]). Soldiers with machine guns walked up and down. One stopped, shoving his piece around his back so he could lift a little child high enough to pick fruit from a tree. An elegant backpacker, Audrey Hepburn–style European, looked intently into the restaurant stand as she walked up the hill from the boat. Cipher asked her what she was looking for, and she gave him a name. He told her the guy wasn't around, then told me she was looking for the guy who loved to suck pussy. Two young German women with delicate faces walked in a loose embrace up the street. They looked expectant and a little sad, like two angels from *The Wings of Desire,* Wim Wenders' film about an angel who longs to exist in time, to enter history.

Having escaped the mythic cocoons holding their mundane realities in place, European travelers ride to places like Livingston on the impulse to break out, to realize suppressed potentialities and desires. And the folks in Livingston are ready to receive them, projecting sexualized tropical fantasies advertised through word of mouth and tourist brochures. Mythic interplay is the motive of history, guiding the destiny of human bodies and their parasites. But then again, perhaps the notion that myth guides history is naive. For on some level we enter into myths willingly, in both the mundane and transgressive variants. We agree to keep silent about the active nature of our participation, acting as if mythic illusions take us by surprise, or are stronger than our complicities in the arrangements of power. But if they were, the larger political economic structures that separate the majority of folk who jet to the tropics from the majority of those who live there would dissolve, and some progress toward egalitarianism might take place in some small niches of the tourist industry. This, we know, does not happen, even in the small yet proliferating niches created by "eco"-tourism. We are back, then, to sex and money.

Near one of the quieter bar-restaurants, a pretty blond woman and a little girl of about five strolled along the beach holding hands. The woman wore a wraparound cloth leaving her shoulders bare, and the little girl's dress was hiked up, her nakedness bare to sunlight and stares. A local man told Cipher that the woman had asked about a nude beach, which he took as an open invitation to have intercourse. I talked to her. She seemed to be an intelligent, hip California type getting carried away by the place and especially the Garifuna men. (She was not alone in this. White women came from all over the world to test the sexual waters of Livingston.) She was thinking about throwing everything over back home and moving down. But she had a lot to straighten out—her career as a family counselor, two houses, a divorced father with partial custody of her child, etc. We laughed at the impossibility of it all. I couldn't help but like her lighthearted fuck-it-all attitude at the same time that I worried about her recklessness and hoped she got the men to use condoms.

That night Cipher and I were dancing in a disco that didn't especially attract tourists. We were dancing with our daypacks on. Three soldiers ordered us off the floor, out into the dark silence of the beach. Their flashlights and machine guns pointed to the sand, where we dumped out the contents of our packs. The vegetables that we had bought at the market tumbled out. We had no marijuana. They let us go.

The U.S. government has been encouraging Guatemalans to be vigilant soldiers in the drug war, assuring them the resources they need to continue terrorizing the people more generally. Tourists, anthropologists, and missionaries are generally immune from this sort of harassment, but if they stray from appropriate illegal behaviors in designated areas, or challenge military power in any way, they are susceptible to the same violence as ordinary citizens. I had given myself some leeway in terms of my involvements in local events. Dropping the professional stranger's guise created a vulnerability that I wouldn't have ordinarily assumed. In return, I had access to a level of local understanding that would otherwise be hidden.

One morning walking in the shallows along the beach, we espied her again: The tall one in woman's clothes was hauling in the fishing net with the men.

The Dream Before (for Walter Benjamin)
a song by Laurie Anderson from *Strange Angels*[1]

Hansel and Gretel are alive and well
and they're living in Berlin.
She's a cocktail waitress.
He had a part in a Fassbinder film.
And they sit around at night now
drinking schnapps and gin.
And she says: Hansel, you're really bringing me down.
And he says: Gretel, you can really be a bitch.
He says: I've wasted my life on our stupid legend.
When my one and only love was the wicked witch.

She said: What is history?
And he said: History is an angel
being blown backward into the future.
He said: History is a pile of debris.
And the angel wants to go back and fix things,
to repair things that have been broken.
But there is a storm blowing in Paradise,
and the storm keeps blowing the angel
backwards into the future.
And this storm,
this storm is called Progress.

The famous children have fallen out of their fairy tale. No longer
the mythic vehicles of innocence conquering evil: Gretel, the witch-
killer, is a waitress, Hansel is an out-of-work actor yearning for the
dead witch. Diffused through the postwar wreckage of Berlin, evil is
no longer made coherent by the figure of the witch. Without her, the

The lyrics of "The Dream Before" are reprinted with permission of Canal Street Com-
munications/E.T.C. from *Strange Angels* © 1989 by Warner Brothers

angel is transfixed by diffuse anxiety and alienation. She's rendered motionless as the winds of progress push her backward into the future. Incapable, she can't restore life to the dead or reason to the destroyed. I can easily imagine Hansel and Gretel drinking beer and smoking pot in an outdoor Livingston bar, an invisible angel looking on helplessly as Hansel, worried but weak in his cups, watches Gretel being seduced by a local man of dubious distinction.

We Met at the Cross of Love Cantina

Public events like Easter in Livingston, which bring together regional people from Guatemala, Belize, and Honduras with visitors from North America and Europe, represent an immense opportunity for HIV. Given the epidemic's global reach, some among the thousands who had unprotected sex during the celebration were bound to have returned to their daily routines infected, unintentionally ramifying into new local networks of potential HIV transmission. By Easter of 1990, when I visited Livingston, there were 176 official AIDS cases in Guatemala; by 1997, the figure jumped to 1,787, a tenfold increase (WHO 1991, 1997).

I do not believe that there is any way to count the possibilities for infection associated with the carnivalesque context. There are just too many brief, randomized sexual encounters among people in festive and intoxicated states. This ritual universe defies categorical attempts to order it. Devising an intervention, whether by government, artists, or activists seems almost folly. Episodic, sexually inflected celebrations such as these encourage fatalism: The death end of Easter looms larger than the rebirth. The question of viral explosion remains unthinkable.

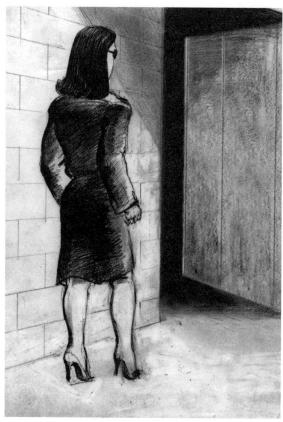

Marilyn Tan heading down alley.

PART III Crime

A bat at sundown
glides, silently seeking
other sundowners.

— *C. Jason Dotson*

9 / Desperate

You don't go down with a hard, short fall—you just sort of shuffle along
And loosen your load of the moral code, till you can't tell the right from the wrong.

— *Clarence Leonard Hay*[1]

We would like to believe that people who know that they are HIV-positive and understand how HIV is transmitted would do all in their power to avoid infecting others. This belief underlies public health and civil rights thinking about the reasonableness of keeping the identity of those who are infected private. That people mean well and have the wherewithal to protect themselves and others is a belief, not a fact. We really don't have empirical evidence that it is true. What's more, we know it is still common for people to engage in unprotected sex and shoot drugs with used needles, and like all humans, some of them are in the habit of showing extreme disregard for the well-being of their intimates, associates, and customers.

After all, government-approved businesses that collect and sell blood products around the world have shown that they are capable of extreme disregard for the lives of their customers. In Canada, Germany, Japan, and England, top executives of national blood companies have been convicted for HIV-related decisions that erred on the side of greed rather than caution. Hemophiliacs and their families in the United States have so far been unsuccessful in making decision makers publicly accountable for infecting 80 percent of those who received HIV-tainted factor (anti-hemophilia blood coagulation factor concentrate) between 1980 and 1985. During this period, the CDC had warned the Red Cross that there was evidence that an unknown fatal organism may be transmitted through blood and that it would be prudent to track it with the test for hepatitis B. But the Red Cross didn't use the hepatitis B test. It was too expensive. Scientific evidence had not yet solidified to their satisfaction (HIV had not yet been identified). They also chose not to warn any of their customers that the expensive blood products, which presumably would extend their lives, might in fact kill them. Hemophiliacs who have filed suit within the United States are convinced that by January 1983 the manufacturers of factor should have fully understood the risks involved. They argue that manufacturers should have taken steps to ensure the safety of blood products and, at the very least, should have warned hemophiliacs of the dangers *before* March 1985, when they began screening all blood for HIV (Shilts 1987, Andersen 1994).[2]

The point is, prostitutes, junkies, and other people "in the life" don't have a corner on knowingly or intentionally putting other people at risk of HIV infection. Scientists, doctors, and executives who have great responsibilities and who have received the highest rewards are capable of being reckless with our fate, causing widespread damage as a result. At least most prostitutes and junkies have had the kind of hard-luck lives that you could believe might generate occasional depravity. They don't seem nearly as evil as some spoon-fed white collar types. Don't you agree?

Back to the life. . . .

T h e r e ' s   N o t h i n g   G o i n g   O n   i n   I o w a

There was that initial feeling of disconcertedness that accompanied my search for the Adam's apple, sign of the biological male. She came into the northside field station in Chicago with an old Italian man. They were homeless and did not meet official AIDS project criteria, but I paid her for an informal interview. Her description of the chaos, violence, and unpredictability of her life and the lives of those whom she was close to underscores how people who are sick, poverty-stricken, and narcotized might not even begin to struggle with the practical and ethical aspects of controlling the transmission of HIV between themselves and others.

■ She said she still felt a bit faint. A trick hit her with a tire iron and she got twenty-seven stitches. I couldn't see them, she said, because they were under her wig. She said she hadn't had a bath in over a month, since her man ran off with the money. She found him again and now they wanted to try and stick together. She turned a trick to get three dollars so she could go to a clinic. She wasn't feeling well (the other seventeen dollars out of the twenty she earned went for cocaine). But she didn't really abuse drugs as much as alcohol. She just wanted to get off the cold streets.

The other day she stabbed her lover, the Italian man, and then he went to jail. They were doing cocaine. She was in the bathroom, in a confined space and he came in. The people in the apartment they'd been staying in egged her on. The two of them had been sleeping on a little couch. The woman there made her do housework in the day and sent her out to trick at night.

The people in the apartment egged her on. She was just poking at her man with the knife. Then they lay down together and made up and all of a sudden he rolled over. He had internal wounds. He was lying over the coffee table and his (other) girlfriend kicked him. Then he shat

133

his pants. So Stitches was there wiping his ass and there were all these stab wounds. Paramedics came and took him to jail.

Stitches used to be a nurse. She got her degree at the University of Iowa in 1972. She worked as a nurse for six years. She started doing Red Devils (Seconals) around 1968. She was shooting dope and working in a strip joint two years after she got her degree. She said that a guy called Uncle John put her on to it and a lesbian put a needle in her arm.

Stitches taught her girlfriend how to turn tricks and her girlfriend got AIDS. They sent her back to Iowa. Girlfriend was crying and crying. But she came back to Chicago to die. There's nothing going on in Iowa.

She was a walking skeleton. And as of this day, she was still out there turning tricks.

I wonder how many story fragments like this appear in the field notes of researches on AIDS intervention projects across the United States, stories that fall between the proscribed categories of analysis, anomalies that worry the field worker just until the next tragedy is told. I don't think it even occurred to me the day I spoke to Stitches that it would be prudent for me to try to find and help Stitches' friend. It wasn't in my job description.

Perpetrator or Victim?

"I'm sick of sex."   —*Deborah Johnson*

Officer Jennings watched the vehicle in the alley turn its lights off and back in behind an abandoned building. It was March 27, 1993, at 20:00 hours at the corner of Fifth and Martin Luther King in Lexington, Kentucky. Jennings drove slowly by the vehicle and saw a white woman duck down in the passenger seat. Jennings turned around on Fourth Street and saw the vehicle leaving hurriedly on Fifth. It was Deborah Johnson, a woman known to the police: She had been arrested for prostitution six times in the last three years and was a documented and informed HIV-positive. After advisement, Kenneth Ross, the man who was driving the car, reported that Johnson offered him oral sex for twenty dollars. Ross witnessed Officer Jennings's post-arrest complaint, which charged Johnson with "procuring another, prostitution to commit* with knowledge of HIV infection." She was eventually convicted of more traditional charges— wanton endangerment, first degree, and terroristic threats.[3]

She was sentenced to a year in the county jail and didn't make headlines in Lexington until six months later. The television and newspaper reporters met Johnson when they went to the jail to interview inmates who intentionally committed crimes to be jailed so that they could receive free medical treatment. But Johnson didn't mean to get arrested. Indeed, Johnson told a reporter how she spent the previous three years trying to infect hundreds of men while working the city's streets.

■ The men that I dated, I wanted them to catch it. I had been beat up and cut up and raped so many times by different men. I wanted to pay these men back. When I got out of their car, I'd laugh. "I struck again, I got this one! Ha, ha!!!"

The front-page headline read "Ex-Lexington prostitute says she tried to transmit HIV."

That Johnson had a lousy life is no surprise. She told the reporter that she ran away from home at fourteen and had been shooting cocaine since she was seventeen. At twenty-six, she had an epileptic fit and learned she was HIV-positive from the blood test. While still a young woman, Johnson said that two Mexican men once raped her in Houston. Now years later, she wants revenge. If a Mexican man buys her sexual services she'd try and infect him.[4] The rapists had forced her to have anal sex, and now if anyone asks for it, she'll insist on another penetrative mode and then try to give her customer the virus just for asking. Then there are those with beards, or those who looked mean and cold-hearted. She'd be happy not to use condoms with them.

The newspaper includes enough information about Johnson's background that she becomes an ambivalent figure. Penned in by bad luck and evil intent, she is poised at the paradoxical intersection of victim and perpetrator of crime—someone who has experienced violence and looks forward to an early death and someone who wants to take as many people down with her as she can.[5] (She did express some remorse for the wives and children of her customers.)

In contrast, the prostitutes who worked the stroll with her didn't stress ambivalence. They told reporters that they had even tried to warn her customers that she was infected. Johnson said she always managed to slough it off, telling the johns that the other girls were "just jealous because you picked me up and not them." The johns must have wanted sex real bad.

Public health professionals took the media event as an opportunity for education, as well they might. To the left side of the front page headline, over a quote about how happy Johnson was to try and infect men, was Johnson's picture, a plain woman with short hair and glasses. On the right side was a shaded sidebar called "Testing recommended," calling for all who had sex with Johnson to get tested, and anyone else who had concerns, assuring that test results would remain anonymous. The article continued on page 8, the text accompanied by two information-filled sections on "Factors affecting infection" and "No charges pending." The latter explained that unless a client-victim came forward to say that they had sex with Johnson, the prosecutor could not use the new 1992 state law that makes it a felony for any person to commit, offer, or agree to commit prostitution by engaging in sexual activity when he or she knew or had been informed that he or she could possibly transmit the virus through sexual activity. Without at least one client, the prosecutors couldn't begin to put a case together.

About five months after her public debut, Johnson hit the news-paper again, though she no longer merited placement on the front page. She was involved in an altercation with a fellow inmate, con-victed murderer LaFonda Fay Foster.[6]

One spring night in 1986, Foster and another white woman went on a three-hour rampage. They tore through Lexington, stabbing, shooting, running people over with a car, and setting them on fire. They killed five. Foster was sentenced to the electric chair in 1987. Ken-tucky had no death row for women, so she was sent to Oklahoma City. In 1991, the Kentucky Supreme Court overturned Foster's death sen-tence, and Foster was sent back to the Fayette County Jail to await re-sentencing. In 1992, a jail officer resigned after having been accused of sexual contact with Foster. In 1994, Foster had a blowup with Johnson.

Apparently Johnson came to disagree with the Supreme Court's decision to overturn Foster's death sentence. So one day when they were returning to their cells from recreation hour in the day room, Johnson called Foster a whore and said that she'd make sure that Foster got the death penalty this time. Not to be outdone, Foster threatened to have Johnson and her family killed. Afterwards, John-son admitted to dripping blood into Foster's coffee to try and infect her with HIV.

Johnson boldly offers a macabre service: If the state won't use its powers to strap this multiple murderess into an electric chair, Johnson will kill her with a slower, less sure, but available method. She tried to use infected blood as a weapon. The idea is horrifying, but in this case, the victim inspires little sympathy. As a jailer told the reporter, the two women are suited to each other. But Johnson's crime elicits a more disturbing comparison; that is, the logic of retri-bution that underlies her act is consistent with the logic of the death penalty. To me, the *form* of Johnson's perversity is less frightening than this logical coincidence.

Jacqui, the first prostitute I interviewed in Chicago, who worked in the great divide along the southern border of the University of

Chicago campus, wanted the woman whom she knew to be HIV-positive to get off the stroll. She knew that the HIV-positive worker could infect the customers who frequented the stroll and, through the customers, herself as well. Perhaps the infected woman continued to work sex because it was the only way she knew how to survive, like Stitches' dying friend from Iowa who worked the northside. Perhaps, like Johnson, she acted with malicious intent, trying to infect the men who bought sex from her, and recklessly disregarding the lives of her coworkers and her customer's wives and children. But I'd hazard a guess that the explanations about why the HIV-infected woman continued to put her at risk would not make much of a difference to Jacqui. She just wanted her to stop working. Explanations of bad acts contribute to understanding, but they do not justify them.

With a Gun and a Rumor

Using HIV as a weapon is not strictly a biological event; that is, it doesn't necessarily involve viral transmission between physical bodies. Symbolic use of HIV as a weapon is key to understanding the public's impulse for criminalization. In the case that follows, a man kills seven people. The use of "AIDS" in a verbal assault was just one of an escalating assortment of terrors confronting his principal victim, a woman he "loved." Like ex-prostitute Johnson, the murderer had a lousy life, most of it on the wrong side of the law. Like her, he aimed to carry out his deed by any means necessary.

Spat out of an overcrowded prison with little or no money, Darnell Collins returned to the casino-encrusted ghetto town of his childhood. The destructive powers possessing his spirit led to the events reported on the front page of the *New York Times* Metro Section late one June:[7]

> He took the Muslim name, Mwanza, but never did have the faith. Ten years in prison put him off balance. He killed

the woman he loved along with her mother, his drug dealer, and four random victims in New York City. He was fatally shot by the local police in Nutley, New Jersey, June 21, 1995.

He came from Atlantic City, Drug City, where the burned-out, boarded up streets lead right up to the grand limousine-choked entrances of the oceanfront casinos. His father was killed in Vietnam and by 9, Collins was in reform school for assault, shoplifting, larceny, attempted arson, trespassing and general "incorrigibility." It went on till he got 15 years in prison for holding up a candy store with a cap gun (i.e., robbery, aggravated assault, and violation of probation). In 1990, he got another seven for stabbing a fellow inmate in Rahway State.

His barber said Collins bragged that he had stabbed someone 23 times with a sharpened toothbrush in the shower, keeping notes on how it went in his Assassination Book. He was repeatedly denied parole, but in 1994, after 11 months of good behavior, the board released him.

He had a violent edge, said the men in the park. But he was determined to stay out of prison, get a life, spend time with his two sons. He was a good dancer, a light-skinned girl's man with a trimmed goatee. He was easygoing and comfortable with women, said Mr. Black.

He kept losing minimum-wage jobs when the employers learned of his record. He set up curbside, selling incense and posters, buying collages of Nelson Mandela and maps of Africa wholesale in New York City and selling them for $10 to $30 each. He could be generous, giving gifts to friends.

He'd ride his bike over to his mother's rickety three-story wood house and sit on the tilting porch under a shade tree. "Whenever he came here it was a hug and a kiss and hello grandma, even though he knew I was his cousin," said an elderly relative. He met pretty April Gates in the summer of 1994 and it looked like love. She invited him to move into the little white house that she shared with her mother and her 7-year-old son. "He was cute," said the friend who later watched as Collins shot April three times point blank.

He started selling drugs late the same summer they met. It was only a matter of time before he started sampling. April started to pull away and he couldn't take rejection. He smashed the windows of her new gold metallic Saturn on Valentine's Day, according to the first of two restraining orders she obtained. He begged her forgiveness and she dismissed the complaint.

But she wouldn't let him back in the house. He stopped going to New York to buy posters. He started living off handouts. He was rootless in his hometown and she was hoping he would change. When he received the next restraining order, eleven days before the killing, he ripped it up in her face.

"He was strung out over her," said Mr. Black. "I guess he figured if he can't have her, nobody could." He started threatening to kill her. He smashed the windows of her house. He hit her and held a gun to her head. He spread a rumor that April had AIDS so that no one else would take her out.

On June 16th, before the killing began, Collins smoked or injected a quarter ounce of cocaine. "One person can't do that much—it's too much," said Mr. Black. "You want more, more and more, and I'm sure at some point he said to hell with it, I'm going all out."

Stuck in the eye of paranoia, Collins hurled an AIDS rumor into the talk of the town. He tried to turn April Gates into a pariah before he turned her into a corpse. Telling people that she had AIDS, Collins tuned into the political unconscious and used its language as a weapon. AIDS, the master signifier, circulates in a symbolic soup with all the other signs of dread and despair, inseparable from the biological universe where the protein-coated viral body of HIV circulates with pneumonia and syphilis and cancer and toxic waste (to name a few).

AIDS is a resource: a biological weapon for those who want to kill and a symbolic weapon for those content to hate. Like violent television imagery in a society that values free speech: We can't control what people will make of it. What we can do, however, is a better job of helping kids like nine-year-old Collins when his father died, or the older kid who stole some candy and got fifteen years in prison, or the man who was finally released and couldn't get a job, or the man who was taking too much cocaine. Our institutions had plenty of chance to help Darnell, at least they had more responsibility than lone and lovely April. And even after loosing his prison-cultivated fury upon the poor community from whence he came, the state's attempts to protect April with a piece of paper were feeble. But why didn't she insist on his arrest after he threatened to kill her, hit her, smashed her windows, and held a gun to her head? And why did the community folks act as mere spectators?

Once desperation sets in, we can't control the riptides in the AIDS unconscious. For people like Collins and Johnson, we need to provide love, education, and economic opportunities in their youth, and not leave them to the prisons and the strolls. If we did, I bet we'd stop seeing these kinds of stories in the newspapers. Until we do, many "innocent victims" will continue to bear the brunt of our collective failures.

Rights and Wrongs

Laws become described and enforced in the spirit of our prejudices.

— *Patricia Williams*

Anything said or done about AIDS that does not give precedence to the knowledge, the needs, and the demands of people living with AIDS must be condemned.

— *Douglas Crimp*

CRIME

The stigma of being HIV-positive is a cultural force. Like prostitution, drug addiction, and homosexuality, the label can be powerfully negative. Not only do the blood test results mean that you will probably die a more painful, earlier death than you'd hoped, but if you want to continue to live life openly and honestly, you end up having to deal with everyone else's terror of disease; and in order to protect others, you may have to deny yourself some cherished intimacies. Like racism, being HIV-positive can cause one to lose one's life chances, independent of one's strength and intellect. For some people this means watching taken-for-granted privileges evaporate; basic necessities like housing, medical insurance, and employment suddenly denied or withdrawn. For people barely surviving at the margins, accustomed to the unreliability of basic necessities, being HIV-positive may be just one more blow in a mounting series.[8]

But secrecy is HIV's muse. At the same time that privacy and confidentiality guarantees protect HIV-positive people from abuse by intimates,[9] neighbors, coworkers, insurance companies, and landlords, secrecy is bound tightly to sexual risk, inhibiting some sexual partners from negotiating prevention techniques and public health workers from using knowledge of serostatus and risk activity to warn people who are likely to be, or may have been, exposed.[10] The principals of privacy and confidentiality guiding AIDS policy have provided a foundation for public trust in medical testing and treatment even as they have helped fight injustice in the culture wars. But when it comes to dealing with individual bad actors, these principals can sometimes function as barriers to prevention.

Criminality does not protect you from AIDS, and it is unlikely that getting AIDS transforms people of bad character into angels before they die. Believing that people are rational beings who have the spiritual and material resources to act for the greater good and the wherewithal to protect themselves and others from the virus is an act of faith. Like a mantra, a rights-oriented public health chant may calm fears of unbridled discrimination, but like that other potentially positive act—making love—it may in some cases increase vulner-ability. Whose discrimination and whose lovemaking are at issue? There is no level playing field. Departing from a belief in human rationality and goodness is a risk easier for some folk to assume than others. If you are labeled as a criminal in one sphere of activity, it tends to make you a suspect in others. State coercion is unequally distributed, layered law upon law, decision upon decision, so that certain classes of persons, such as prostitutes, are always the first to lose their rights (Bergman 1988).

Questions and answers chase round my head: Dare we look to the criminal law to help solve problems caused or exacerbated by disease? (A scary thought . . . abuses associated with the drug war suggest not.) But should drug war abuses distort public faith that the criminal law can ever be used for good purpose? (No, but nor can we be naive about what laws accomplish, even when they are enacted in good faith.) Is it in any case possible to distinguish the few HIV-positive people who have malign intent without persecuting the many who are peaceful and caring? (In some cases, yes.) Does intention make a difference once an infection occurs? (It does to some people.) What about cases of repeated intentional infection in spite of public health warning? (At the individual level, it makes sense to legally intervene, but such action may have minimal or negative effect at the population level.) Is it possible to avoid unequal enforcement of criminal HIV laws so that white-collar criminals and prostitutes, heteros and gays, rich and poor, get the same treatment? (Not yet.) Are there better ways of getting HIV-positive prostitutes off the streets than putting them in jail and prison? (Sure.) What about the violent and the insane? (I think not!)

Quiet Riot

The stories in this chapter so far have focused on people who have used HIV as a weapon either physically or symbolically. The stories are tied together by the marginality of their personal histories. Stitches' friend Deborah Johnson and Darnell Collins are stuck on the wrong side of the law. They don't step out of beautiful lives and suddenly do something crazy. Instead, their victims have the bad luck of crossing into the danger zones of their terrible lives.

The final story in this chapter is also about people with marginal histories who resort to using HIV as a weapon. It is unusual in that it involves a marginalized group of people who, acting in concert, use themselves as their own victims. They represent their communal suicidal act as political resistance, a notion that is not diminished by, but must be related to, their extraordinary youth and their cultural locale.

The youths in question refused to follow the rules of Castro's Cuba. They were harassed by police for crimes of style, a collective enterprise at the core of subcultural group identity (Hebdige 1988; Ferrell 1996). Self-inoculation with HIV-infected blood and self-imposed retirement to sanitoria seem like excessive responses to police harassment and economic strain. At the time the youth chose to become infected, the sanitoria were like prisons—albeit with guaranteed medical care, good food, and television. The documentary *Al Margen del Margen* (Beyond Outcasts) dramatizes the way in which HIV-infected residents in the sanitoria were made to feel like criminals. They had little choice but to stay on the grounds, isolated from their friends, families, and work. Contrary to official representation of the facilities as a humane and pragmatic response to the island's AIDS epidemic, gay residents felt that their forced retirement was an extension of the repressive anti-homosexual campaigns of the Cuban revolution, and the youth felt it as discrimination against "irresponsible" youth more generally.[11]

But one group of youths took this rebuke as a challenge. Here is the story: Sometimes a nihilistic idea occurs to one or more persons in a subcultural group and it seems like a logical solution to a dilemma. Apparently, based on the pieces about them in the *Sunday New York Times Magazine* and on *National Public Radio,* that's what happened to the Rockers.[12] Identity and protest were the mobilizing issues, expressed in musical taste and personal style. Led Zeppelin was their band of all bands; Black Sabbath and Rush were also cool. Later in the eighties the Rockers turned to Iron Maiden, Quiet Riot, Guns 'n' Roses, Anthrax, and Megadeath. Rockers wore black and leather as much as possible; wristbands with metal spikes or studs, earrings, crucifixes, and combat boots. They didn't pick fights, paint graffiti, or start fires. They had long and tangled hair, wore ripped jeans, and liked bandannas and T-shirts printed with the U.S. flag. They sometimes swallowed or injected prescription drugs.

The police didn't like them because they wanted to live by different rules. Youth who dressed like Rockers were beaten, fined, imprisoned, and forced into the military. But Rockers would not relent, and one day, according to Rocker legend, a handful decided to inject themselves with HIV-infected blood donated by friends. They vowed slow suicide at state expense. A protest it would be, if they got enough attention. The process was simple: Get a needle. Visit an infected friend or other willing donor. Extract the infected blood and release the charge into your own arm. For some, the injection was a freeing act; seroconversion took only weeks.

> The number of self-infected
> Rockers? Who knows for sure,
> a hundred, may be more.
> With a cohort of young
> women who could not part
> from the infected boys
> who stole into their hearts.

One youth injected himself in his home province at fifteen years of age. The police had been hassling him with beatings and fines. He couldn't take it anymore and decided to inject. Another troubled by police made it all the way to twenty, the year he got engaged. He

CRIME

failed to get infected when he went to a town known for its high
AIDS rate. He eventually succeeded back home, where he got infected
blood from a friend.

> His fiancé knew he injected
> himself, but she wanted to stick
> by him. They went ahead with unsafe
> sex and she too became a victim.
> Now, like almost all the women
> that folly she too regretted.

The circulation of AIDS stigma in the political unconscious is telling and ironic. First, people who are infected with HIV are locked up
in sanitoria as if they are dangerous criminals, even when there is no
evidence that particular individuals would ever do anything to hurt
anyone through recklessness or maliciousness. Then, young people
who are clearly not dangerous criminals are nevertheless harassed by
police as if they are, until in response, the young people purposefully
become infected so that they could stay at the sanitaria!

As it happened, the Rockers are Cubans, and their suicidal acts
cannot be separated from national and international battles for the
body, soul, and economy of Cuba. But in contrast to media representation, I don't believe the event is inextricably linked to Castro's
dictatorial rule. I believe that things like this could happen anywhere
in the nineties where youth felt that they had no chance to be happy
and free.

Sometimes being happy and free entails a test of fate. For example, Emily Martin (1994, 236) cites the case of five Texas girls who
had sex with an HIV-infected male to get into a gang (Associated Press
1993). If the test came up negative, then it reportedly proved to the
gang that they were brave and tough enough to have unprotected sex
and that their physical body was tough enough to fight the disease.
The Texans' aim was not to get infected, as was the Rockers, but the

spirit of challenge motivating their intentional encounters with HIV are not dissimilar.

> The virus enters language through routes littered with despair.
> Embodied in youth's rebellion,
> *Cuidado* all! Take care!

10 / The Positively Arrogant Mishap

I met Liz Locke in Bloomington, Indiana, in 1993, the night she first told me this story, the year that Q died. Her story is a marked reversal of the stories from the previous chapter. The sense of malign neglect that runs through the lives of Stitches' HIV-positive friend, Deborah Johnson, and Darnell Collins is dispelled. There are no police, guns, jails, or prisons. It is a story about a coherent community, not colliding individuals in an alienating and confusing world. And unlike the Cuban Rockers, the people of Liz's story live in a privileged world, where meditative souls engaged in creative work, building a sacred and economically successful community by practicing ancient principals in a contemporary setting. But then came AIDS, and almost everything changed. The moral authority of the highest leaders was thrown into question, and the community's peace and stability exploded. If the fluids are right, the virus does not distinguish between oppression and sacredness. Mindlessly moving from body to body, the virus has no notion of the havoc it causes.

Some months after we met, Liz agreed to record a full account on tape; I write from the transcript and our continuing conversation.

An earlier version of this chapter entitled "Sacred Deviance and AIDS in a North American Buddhist Community" appeared in *Law and Policy* 16(July 1994): 323–40, and is used here by permission of Blackwell Publishers.

Sacred Deviance

Taking a vow of refuge is like getting into your own boat. Every-
body is in their own boat on this vast, limitless, profound
ocean of life. And every human being, every sentient being
is in their own boat. We're all out there, alone together. And
the refuge is that there is no refuge. This is as safe as it gets:
alone, in a little rowboat, on a vast ocean. It's not very com-
forting. . . . [laugh]

Liz arrived at the Vajradhatu International Buddhist Church in
Boulder, Colorado, in 1976, when she was nineteen, with the intention of staying two weeks to visit her brother. She had no desire to
get involved (again) in another imported Asian religion. Indeed, if it
wasn't Walt Whitman, she said, she didn't want anything to do with
it. But in those two weeks she met Trungpa Rinpoche:

■   I was working on what was to become the main headquarters of
the church, a building called Dorje Dzong (Indestructible Fortress) in
Boulder. We were transforming it from an old office building to the
main shrine room and offices. And I had been given a screwdriver with
a piece of sandpaper wrapped around the end and I had been told
to get the paint off the newel post at the foot of the stairs, which had
all these curlicues and carvings and it had six coats of paint on it. And
I had been working on this goddamn newel post for about two hours
with the little piece of sandpaper and the screwdriver and the whole
time my thought process was getting speedier and speedier and angrier and angrier and I wanted nothing to do with these people and
what am I doing here with this goddam screwdriver anyway and I had
just gotten to the point where I had decided to drive the screwdriver
through. . . . Oh, no, an announcement came down that Rinpoche had
changed his mind. Everything was going to be painted white and as a

result we didn't have to remove the paint now. Now this is classic in a Tibetan tradition, in any Buddhist tradition, it's like I told you to do it this way, but now I want you to do it that way. Just to screw up your plans. So my response to that was that I was going to drive the screwdriver through the newel post and I had my hand raised and I looked around and everybody else was standing very quietly with their hands behind their backs and I thought what the fuck is going on here? And I looked to the doorway, and there's this little Asian guy in a suit with two other Anglo guys in suits standing behind him, sort of holding him up, and everybody is looking at him like he's the main show. And I didn't know that it was Trungpa Rinpoche. But I'm standing there with the screwdriver aimed at the newel post [laugh], and I looked at him and he looked at me, and all of a sudden I was busily back working on the newel post, with no thought having gone through my mind whatsoever. Except, Oh, that's what I'm doing here. I mean, I didn't know who this guy was, until afterwards. But it was this little smile on his face. He looked at me. And my response to me was, Oh, I get it. And I went right back to work. So we can add this up to my state of mind, or we can say that this actually was the Buddha in person, which is what I came to see it as.

Chögyam Trungpa Rinpoche was the eleventh incarnation of Trungpa Tulku of the Kagyu lineage, head of ancient Tibetan monasteries abandoned to Chinese invaders in the 1950s. He carried his teachings into the world, establishing communities in Scotland, the United States, Japan, Germany, England, and Canada. By the mideighties, interlocking (mainly male) hierarchies administered his approach to the path of enlightenment for between three and five thousand followers.[1]

When he first got to Boulder, as the story goes, Rinpoche was living in a house in the canyons. People would sit around at the foot of his bed and listen to him teach and tell stories and he'd drop acid with them once in a while. It was much more loose. But after His

Holiness Karmapa came and hipped everybody to who they were dealing with, everything changed. This tremendous sense of formality crept into everything. Because they had never met anybody like Karmapa before, and Karmapa came saying "Do you know who this is?" And they all went, "Oh my God, and we've been like slapping him on the back and hanging out and drinking coffee with him and stuff." So people stood up straighter and wore better clothes and were much more formal and everything changed. By the 1980s, it was a very stratified society.

In 1979, three years after she joined the community, Liz took her vow of refuge. She remained a member for another seven years. She was not on the Board of Directors, nor was she one of the women students selected to sexually service Rinpoche and his inner court. She was one of the hundreds of members of the community who were fully integrated into the white, middle-class, tax-paying upwardly mobile world of the town. The members ran schools open to all, including a preschool, an elementary school, and Naropa Institute, an accredited college. They ran a newspaper with international distribution (the *Vajradhatu Sun*) and a private press to publish Trungpa Rinpoche's talks. Members ran departments of practice, health, and social well-being, as well as a credit union, and those who were bar-certified lawyers formed an arbitration board to provide legal advice in matters such as divorce disputes. Their mission was to handle disputes according to Buddhist principles of compassion. A military-style force, peaceful warriors called *kasung*, wore khakis and walkie-talkies and protected Rinpoche, his followers, and the Teachings. Enlightenment was the ultimate goal of all their activities.

Known as Tantric Buddhism in the West, theirs was "the mishap lineage," called this because its students tended to come upon it through accident or misfortune. It began with the birth of Shakyamuni in the sixth century B.C.E. In the mishap lineage, acts categorized as deviant by conventional standards might be acts that, when mindfully carried out, enable the greatest possibility of transcendence.

As long as you sustain a disciplined focus on the emptiness at the center of existence and a compassion for all sentient beings, you can reach the limits of human experience.

This devotional path requires cosmic outrageousness. Sit at the feet of scurrilous men who live with wild dogs, prostitutes, and rag-men, their teachers said. Eat road kill. Love and annihilate the body, individual and social. One guy Liz knew blew his brains out during a roulette game. The woman he had married three days before watched him die outrageously in the room that night. Some call practitioners of the Kagyu school pigs, but practitioners say at least they won't be born pigs in the next lifetime. They sit like pigs—their quality of discipline is not like Zen Buddhists. It's not "don't move, don't scratch"—the body is a vehicle, and if you need to scratch it you do. Just make sure you're scratching your body and not your mind.

Trungpa Rinpoche was revered by hundreds, perhaps thousands, of North Americans, mostly ex-Catholics and Jews, experimenting with life in the spirit of the time—which included a lot of fucking (gay and straight) and alcohol (reefer and cocaine were not widely used, but they were used, depending on the era and despite the hier-archy's official disapproval of illegal acts). The task was to transmute neurotic addictive clinging to alcohol or drugs into an open, fresh, and generous activity that mirrors the mind, not clouds it. Rinpoche taught how to turn sacred into deviant, deviant into sacred. Like ma-nure is transmuted into crops, vice may be transmuted into virtue. He took his own drinking and sexual activities to extremes by con-ventional standards. Searching for purity is arrogance, he taught, as if the world were too dirty for you. You can't remain unsullied; the more spontaneous you are, the more devoted. Release into sacred-ness, yeah! Killing a flea, loving a friend. Some things have weirder consequences than others. In the cosmic scheme of things, distinc-tions vanish.

Buddhist schools have different ways of understanding the rela-tionship between student and teacher. Some conceptualize it as weaving a fine piece of cloth; for others it involves shaping the cloth into a useful garment that anyone can wear, but in the Tantric tradition, it's like taking the beautiful garment you've woven and tearing it to shreds with a pitchfork. It releases the energy of the garment. Whatever it is that's held back, that separates you from me, self from other, whatever it is that maintains any notion of duality in the world is exploded. However, there is said to be one act that Buddhist schools together single out as something akin to the Christian notion of mortal sin, and that is to kill one's teacher.

Drinking Lessons

In this Tantric tradition, sake (rice wine) is treated as a magical substance that can act as either medicine or poison, depending on the state of the practitioner's mind. One of the elements of living in a first-generation American Buddhist community was that there was a tremendous amount of alcohol consumption and abuse. Sake was the most popular drink. It was used as a religious sacrament, something to be embraced, understood, worked through, and then transformed into a vehicle for further awareness, for becoming awake. Rinpoche used to give what he called drinking lessons. Liz was not advanced enough in the teaching to be involved. The idea was that one remained mindful while one became drunk, noticing each change in consciousness. Rinpoche drank more than anyone Liz had ever known. Somehow he could metabolize the poison into medicine and transform it into a teaching. But by 1980 or 1981, the thing that Liz was becoming the most aware of was that she was terminally alcoholic. No phenomenon has to be rejected, she was told. There is no such thing as alcoholism. It's just a neurotic way of relating to alcohol in which you think there is something out there that has power over you. Meditate, sit, drink mindfully, and then it won't have any power over you.

This teaching was very confusing to her, and it became socially dangerous for her to say, "I'm an alcoholic." Liz found ways to understand the contradictions. One day she asked a visiting teacher: If, as the teachings say, the phenomenal world of the flesh, blood, and stale coffee (*samsara*) is one side of the same coin that being awake is on, how come everyone around here is so busy searching for *nirvana*? He laughed and said: "Of course, they [*samsara* and *nirvana*] have to be together and they are the same thing. But, it's a trick. We say *nirvana* is better because if we didn't, nobody would practice [meditate]." The response satisfied her and helped her to understand the events that were to come.

Some Consequences Are Weirder than Others

She watched as Rinpoche was dying of alcoholism and his inner court pretended nothing was wrong. Trungpa Rinpoche had named Thomas Rich, a gay man from Passaic, New Jersey, to be his dharma heir and lineage holder in 1976. As Osel Tendzin (Radiant Holder of Teachings), Rich was to pass on the teachings to the Vajradhatu community until Rinpoche was reborn: the first Westerner to head a school of Tantric Buddhism. He was an expansive, charismatic man and a great lover of men. It became a mark of prestige for a man, gay or straight, to have sex with the Regent, just as it had been for a woman to have sex with Rinpoche. He was positively arrogant, and, after all, orgasm is one of the rare moments in human life where consciousness is non-dual.

One of the students the Regent had sex with was Q.

Q also had sex with his girlfriend.

Liz had taken a class with the Regent at Naropa Institute, making a strong connection with him:

■ I respected him as my teacher because he was the Regent. He had that position in the community. He had been recognized as Rinpoche's successor, but at the same time, he was an American. He was a lot closer to Walt Whitman than Trungpa Rinpoche, than this Tibetan. And I don't know, because he was a Leo, or because of his style, we had sort of a style in common. I was driving a cab for a good part of that time [late seventies and early eighties] and I was drinking a lot, and I walked with a swagger, and thought I was the toughest bitch on the block basically. And I was told a story once, that I was coming back from the airport, from Denver, wearing my beret in my cab and the Regent and his entourage passed in a limo going in the other direction. And the Regent remarked to one of his *kasung* guards, the driver, "Who is that woman?" They identified me to him, and he said, "Damn classy broad!"

So there was a certain amount of mutual acknowledgment of one another. I was always surprised when it came in my direction. He once referred to me as "my friend" with his arms thrown open in front of many people, which really shocked me. I loved him. I really love him and he was an extraordinary teacher. He could cut to the heart of the matter with no verbiage, or with very little verbiage. He had a poet's heart and he was extremely powerful. That arrogance was such a remarkable knife that he could use it to cut away all the extraneous stuff, whatever was going on, and just walk right into your heart.

But in 1986 Liz formally withdrew her membership. She could not live in a community that continued to deny the phenomenal world a place in its spiritual practice. Trungpa Rinpoche died in April 1987 at the age of forty-seven.

■   You know, if he teaches us, through his drinking, or his death by drinking, fine. But for me, if my body doesn't metabolize alcohol properly, I'm gonna die as a result of this energy. And if you die, you don't get to practice the teachings of the Buddha, because you're dead. So that was the logic I used. And I felt I had to remove myself from the *sangha* (community) per se. Now the reaction to my having left was very strong in some quarters. This was simply not done. You've made a relationship with this teacher. So when I formally left the body of the church, so to speak, it was also formally understood that I had turned my back on Trungpa Rinpoche, that I had broken the student-guru relationship. This was not at all how I felt about the matter. He is my teacher today as we speak. But it was not understood that way, and I became something of a heretic within the community. And heretics within any community are essentially very dangerous people. Because they cause you to doubt what you know. I became — one woman referred to me as a rebel without a cause, that it was my own ego that was making me leave this brilliant, sacred, precious situation. Whatever, it gets very painful. [sigh]

Around this same time, in the mid-1980s, the Regent had learned that he was infected with HIV.

The community's most influential doctor and its board of directors knew that the Regent was infected. They kept the information in confidence. None spoke about the Regent's HIV infection or even about AIDS prevention more generally. They felt that articulating these concerns threatened the integrity of the community. They feared being caught by the ugly political unconscious of AIDS, being transformed in the public imagination from a handsome and talented tax base into a sex and drug-crazed cult (as did happen to Rajneesh's community in Oregon). Bolstered by their beliefs and tied to their economic successes, the doctor and the board sacrificed the lives of students. None of the persons privileged to understand the implications of having sex with the Regent uttered any warnings to the men who had sex with him, or to any of the greater numbers of others with whom the students had sex in turn. The community was kept in the dark as effectively as the hemophiliacs were kept in the dark by the blood banks. But unlike the decisions that U.S. blood bank executives made between 1983 and 1985, the doctor's and the board's decision was made well after HIV had been identified and North

Americans had begun to acknowledge the gruesome implications of
the epidemic.

The Regent got pneumonia in the summer of 1988.

The expansive man who loved to eat, drink, and smoke, suddenly
quit smoking and went on a macrobiotic diet. Whispers that the Regent might have AIDS were dismissed as impossible. The people
would not allow the man to be human, he held out hope for
enlightenment.

Q let it be known that he was infected with HIV in December of
that year. A self-identified heterosexual, Q identified the Regent as
the only possible source of infection. Later it was revealed that transmission must have occurred when he gave the Regent blow jobs, and
may have occurred as a result of a single blow job. (According to
current epidemiological evidence, this is a highly unlikely, but not
impossible.)

Then Q's girlfriend became infected.

The news whipped through the global Tantric Buddhist networks, sparking paranoia of mythic proportions. Liz wondered if
she'd thrown her life away to a cosmic criminal. Has this just turned
into a joke life?

The inner court believed that they were spiritually bound to con-
ceal the knowledge of the Regent's serostatus. This provided a useful
alibi for the second reason they had; that is, that they were materially
bound to a lavish status quo. Liz tells how she felt when she heard the
news of Q:

■   So there was unprotected sex. And the horrifying part was . . . that
there were five people in the administration of the church, including his
personal physician, who knew that he had been diagnosed five years
earlier as being HIV-positive. And their relationship to him precluded
any possibility that they would ever let it be known outside of their
circle. So they made a choice for the entire community. And that
choice was to believe that his enlightenment would protect everybody

from this illness, which I think is the ultimate act of hubris. I hold those five men as responsible as the Regent. These were people who took it upon themselves to make a decision for everybody, for a thousand people and more. And it was well known how much sex was going on and how incestuous the whole thing was in terms of the whole community. And a virus like AIDS spreads like wildfire in a group of people who are sleeping together to the degree that we were. So I hold them as responsible as I hold him in many ways.

I hold them more responsible in some ways too. And I'll tell you why. Because, the way that I put it for myself is that, if I had somebody beside me in a suit who was there to respond to my every wish for ten years, who stood at my elbow with an ashtray in the event that I should need it, who came to me with my drink on a silver tray with a lace cloth on it in the event that I might be thirsty, and who catered to my every whim for ten years, I might also believe that I was capable of anything. There was a collusion on the part of the community with what I think of as the Regent's deludedness. If you treat somebody like a king, you shouldn't be surprised if they begin to act like one.

Meetings were called in Berkeley and Boulder. Some demanded the Regent resign. He refused. He said that his level of spiritual enlightenment would protect him and his partners from AIDS. A virus might penetrate but not conquer his body or the student body who had given themselves to him in trust. A small group, guided by the Alcoholics Anonymous adage "You are only as sick as your secrets," took the story to the *San Francisco Chronicle*. The Boulder community regarded them as crazy heretics who wanted to destroy the community. Speaking against the teacher was the equivalent of cosmic doom. How dare they criticize someone who was giving them a teaching? To turn one's back on the teacher is akin to killing the teacher, the one cardinal sin.

Q's announcement created turmoil. It was said that the Regent sent spies among them. There were people calling for the Regent's incarceration for murder or for attempted murder. The editorial policy of the *Vajradhatu Sun* newspaper prohibited discussion. Its editor quit.[2] No one called the police; nor did the police call the community.[3] Instead, they turned to community tribunals: Delegations were sent to India and Nepal. The first delegation was more disposed to forgiving the Regent and returned with a message urging kindness and compassion (consistent with the Dalai Lama's pacifism and compassion for the Chinese). A second delegation, determined to transmit the events more fully, returned with a condemnation of the Regent. The elders declared that the Regent had betrayed the student-teacher relationship. Some in Boulder found comfort in this judgment; others dismissed it as foreign influence, too distant from their own experience to be valid.

Discord strained devotion; the community divided. An heiress supported a group who brought the Regent to California and cared for him like royalty until he died, at the age of forty-seven, the same age as Trungpa Rinpoche. A major portion of the Boulder community moved to Halifax, Nova Scotia, to a setting that Rinpoche had established before his death. The monastery in Bhutan sent Rinpoche's son to lead a more sedate, family-oriented scene consistent with chastened times and a more provincial context. Some have stayed on as before; some like Liz, have exiled themselves, living out their vow of refuge without the benefit of community.

On August 28, 1990, the Regent's obituary in the *New York Times* summarized the conflict:

> In December 1988 it became known that Mr. Tendzin's companion had tested positive for the AIDS virus. At a meetings of several hundred Buddhists in Berkeley, California, later that month, Mr. Tendzin acknowledged that he had AIDS and may have infected others.
>
> He said he had known for several years that he was ill but thought he could "change the karma."

Vajradhatu does not prohibit homosexuality or sex with more than one partner. But the issue of Mr. Tendzin's illness split the denomination, with supporters insisting that he remain as head and critics arguing that he must resign because he had betrayed the trust of his followers.

He refused to resign and retained his title, but the church's board took over leadership of the group.

Q died in 1993 in his mid-twenties.

Q's girlfriend is living with HIV.

Liz knows of three other gay men from the community who died of AIDS, but none known to have direct sexual links to the Regent. Members have gotten tested, but the ramifying consequences of these events will probably never be fully discovered.

On December 2, 1993, Liz surfed into this email exchange between one Bear Giles at the University of Colorado and one Lee Rudolph from Clark University, two users of chat groups on new age religion, scientific skeptics, and/or the alternative paranormal:

■ Bear: That reminds me of a local Buddhist leader. I forgot his name; he moved his world headquarters to Canada (Nova Scotia?) a few years ago. . . . Anyway, he caught the HIV virus (and knew it), but continued to have unprotected sex because he believed the purity of him and his flock would protect them. It did not. A fair number of people in Boulder are HIV-positive because of his beliefs.

Lee: I'm blanking on his name—XX Trogyam Rinpoche perhaps? . . . In any case, the story's worse than that. A few years ago, attending a political meeting at a local Quaker meetinghouse, I was thumbing through a magazine someone had left around, which included an exchange of letters on this case (this was after the leader in question was dead). I don't recall whether the claim that "the purity of him and his flock would protect them" was made, or addressed, in that exchange, though it may well have been; what struck me, and stuck in my memory, was that at least one of the writers was making the claim that the leader's transmission of the virus was a deliberate spiritual exercise for the benefit of his followers. (Note: I am not making that claim myself, nor denying it; all I am doing here is reporting— alas, without the ability to cite a specific written source—that someone made that claim, unblushingly, in print. Oh, and the person making the claim seemed to think that the leader was in fact doing a good thing. I cannot agree.)

The sense of outrageousness grows, even as the details of the story fade and Lee Rudolph considers the positive effects of meditation on the immune system. Could there have been *intentional* transmission?

Shoo Fly

Liz told me about how they used to do the shoo fly in Boulder. To get rid of flies in the room, everyone would line up along one end of the room holding up blankets. Walking across in unison, they would shoo the flies outside with blankets so as not to harm them. I have mixed feelings about this. From this perspective, embracing HIV as a sacrament might not be that farfetched. But why didn't the Regent and his healer and decision makers extend their compassion for flies to human devotees?

The tragic events that took place in Boulder's Buddhist community highlight the way in which sacred precepts practiced with the best intentions can precipitate fatal reactions when they combine with a refusal to accommodate to the reality of HIV. The refusal of Catholic hierarchy to allow education about safe sex is prey to the same weakness and will have a much more widespread effect. But the way in which HIV enters into and destroys relatively bounded sexually active communities is a phenomenon that is not necessarily characterized by a contradiction between idealism and pragmatism. For example, a university student told a class on genocide about a little-known catastrophe that happened in her high school: In a county so rural it didn't even boast a town, 110 sexually active students, one-third of the graduating class, became HIV-infected (Phil Parnell, personal communication, Sept. 1996). Similar transmission events have occurred in Brazilian communes (Jean Langdon, personal communication, May 1993).

I am haunted by an image from research past. In 1984, I had just finished a year of fieldwork among the Emberá Indians of Darién, Panama, most of whom live in small, isolated villages and dispersed dwellings along the many rivers that cut through the rain forest (Kane 1994). The Emberá mostly have sex and marry each other, or other Indians of marriageable classes, such as Waunan and Catio. And although there was a community that lived in the slum of Panama City bordering the Canal Zone, most lived upriver. One day I went to the downtown city market with a friend. I was surprised to see four young women whom I'd thought had never been downriver and who had always to my knowledge worn traditional clothes, standing on a corner wearing Western dresses and makeup. Our mutual reaction of embarrassment reinforced my feeling that they were soliciting sex. One of the unintentional consequences of the integration of indigenous peoples into the nation's political economy, I thought at the time. Later, when I got involved in AIDS intervention, I couldn't help worrying that my wild surmise was correct and that the young women might have been infected with HIV from any one of the thousands of sailor-men who came through Panama on freighters or from U.S. or Panamanian soldiers. I couldn't help worrying what would happen if HIV began circulating in the villages. I hope the four young women are healthy and happy and that I worry too much.

11 / Outtakes

Transforming the deviant into the sacred is one thing when carried out in the spirit of enlightenment, quite another when done with malice. The political unconscious of AIDS is a roiling bloody mess. From it arise possibilities for the sickest imaginations. And as suggested by the two stories from Canadian newspapers that I retell here, opportunities to draw on it are not restricted by gender, class, or race. In the two preceding chapters on crime, the misdeeds of the characters are related to systems of oppression or belief. In contrast, the characters presented here are so twisted, they are beyond needing alibis. Their stories should be outtakes, their violence so eccentric that they cannot be used to think through practical problems of law and disease. They're way out there on the bell curve, cracks running deep into the rubble of our AIDS consciousness, where needles lie coated in medical waste and fetuses grow AZT-resistant viruses. The chapter is brief but necessary.

Cocaine Insane

■ Terry Fitzsimmons and Donald Hebert made a suicide pact.[1] Two white men "like a brotherhood of the doomed," said the lawyer who spoke for the defense. Cocaine insane, a three-city rampage ensued. In Montreal they stabbed a cabby several times in the chest. In Toronto they beat their dentist friend to death.

It all started in a Kingston, Ontario, jail, the journalist explains, where Terry was serving time for robbery. A friend of his was stabbed to death; the grapevine told him he was next. So he acted first, stabbing the inmate-killer with a kitchen knife. The next seven years he passed in a Saskatchewan prison solitary cell.

Paroled in '92, Terry served six of his nine years. He settled down in Kingston, Ontario, got married, and impregnated his wife, which is how he left her when he ran off with Don. Don's a man with whom he shared some symbiosis but no sex, said the lawyer for the defense.

Their spree took them to Ottawa on August 4, 1994. After partying through the night, they ended up in an abandoned restaurant. "I can't bear to go to jail for the crimes we have committed," said Don to Terry. Terry then injected himself with two vials of Don's tainted blood, strangled his friend with a T-shirt, then plunged a fifteen-inch butcher blade through his friend's chest.

After washing off Don's blood, Terry went to a phone booth to call 911. He shot more cocaine before getting to the station, to tell police that the killing's got to stop. Terry was disinterested in court procedures, for after all, he said, he'd already sentenced himself. He thought they wouldn't be satisfied with just a prison term. And so he gave them the capital punishment that he thought the good citizens deserved.

Terry tested positive in January 1995.

We tend to think about homicide and suicide in separate behavioral categories, but the Fitzsimmons-Hebert story reveals their overlap. When a man randomly kills a bunch of people, then his friend and himself, the distinction between homicide and suicide impedes understanding: It's all of a piece. Terry Fitzsimmons intentionally injects himself with his friend's HIV-infected blood (a method of administration more efficient than dripping blood in coffee!). Sure to be condemned for multiple murders, he substitutes a penalty of his own devise, implying by his equation that popularity for state-mandated killing is driven by the same blood-thirst as his own. (This despite the fact that there is no death penalty in Canada.) Which is more mad, his or the systemic brutality that brews fury in solitary confinement? Like multiple murderer Darnell Collins (Chapter 8), Fitzsimmons' post-release dementia is fed by toxic doses of injected cocaine. But this madman doesn't get the benefit of insight. Unlike the description of Collins, which set his crime in the context of personal history and community, the brief *Edmonton Journal* article on Fitzsimmons goes no farther back in time than his prison stay. It tells us nothing about his partner Donald Hebert except his serostatus, partnership in crime, and his own untimely death. The story hangs in space. Inexplicable, it must be spit out, undigested and forgotten.

She Ran with High Society, but the Blood Came from a Nobody

Unlike Terry's and Don's trial, which didn't get much press, Marilyn Tan's trial appeared blow by blow.[2] She had a lot more style and money. A demurely sly Tan peered out of the newsprint with her newfound conservative but feminine off-white skirt and jacket ensembles (contrasting with the outfit she wore when she pleaded not guilty nine months before: black miniskirt, with black, white, and hot-pink top and heels). She was a Philippine-born beauty with a taste and talent for multimillionaires. A former model, she had Marilyn Monroe lips, almond-shaped eyes the color of dark chocolate, cheekbones to die for, and an amazing body. . . . She was charged with aggravated assault, conspiracy to administer a noxious substance and administering a noxious substance in relation to HIV attacks on Con Boland. She was also accused of uttering a death threat (to her ex-lover's former girlfriend Jeanette Kunkel, whom she intercepted in an alleyway wearing a black leather trench coat, black stiletto-heeled shoes, and dark glasses, to threaten her with death if she didn't quit seeing Tan's man Boland, whose multimillion-dollar photography business Tan allegedly coveted).

Boland is a celebrated forty-seven-year-old photographer, a portrait specialist, whose subjects have included Pierre Trudeau and Wayne Gretzky. Boland claims that he was twice injected with HIV by his former lover Tan—once in his elegant riverside home in Edmonton and a second time during a sadomasochistic sex session in a California hotel room in June 1992.

Retirees and high school students filled the court for Tan's trial. There hadn't been anything as titillating as this in Alberta, Canada, in a long time. They got an earful:

■ Con Boland told the court he wanted out, but he'd thought he'd at least be nice. No harm in one last fling, she'd said the sex'd be hot. She started as his secretary, but by the night in question, his buttocks were beneath her whip and her ambition was in his business. He wore a jockstrap and clothespins through his nipples. She'd insisted on a blindfold and that he drink hard liquor. After only half a glass he grew ill and fainted. When he awoke his left thigh was bruised. The bruise was admittedly near the whipping, he said in court, though Tan told him at the time that he'd bumped into a dresser. It was only later that he learned how Tan had jabbed him with an AIDS-infected needle.

Their relationship had always been tempestuous. He said she was a spendthrift. She said he was promiscuous and she worried he'd expose them both to AIDS. They continued on together, way longer than they should have. The Crown alleges that the situation drove Tan mad with jealousy and bitterness. They said she wanted Boland dead.

Tan had some conversation with a confidant named Rachel Deitch, who'd voiced a suggestion about an HIV injection that could hurt someone really badly. She tried to take it back, telling Tan that dog feces would work better. But Tan had already figured the logistics. Her sister was a registered nurse in hospitals in California. The tainted blood came from a nobody, and certainly not from work. The sister mailed the vial across to Deitch in Canada, who wrapped it in a Holt Renfrew box and delivered it to Tan.

Deitch tried to tell a doctor, lawyer, and nurse what happened. They thought it was a hoax. She didn't go to the police until Boland launched a lawsuit. Then she tried to get away by telling Boland about Tan.

So he went to get tested, even though he'd been negative nine months before. When he learned of his infection, he went to the police. He admitted in court to shooting cocaine and being partial to hookers, but he swore he always used condoms and nothing but clean needles. Sergeant JoAnn McCartney, officer of vice, testified on his behalf that the prostitutes in Edmonton are a relatively clean lot. In contrast, Tan's lawyer portrayed Boland as an immoral lecher, who must have gotten AIDS from his lifestyle and not Tan's poisonous injection. Boland said he'd only had one STD, then his doctor testified he'd had four.

The judge did not like them (in a trial without a jury). Yes, Tan did go get an AIDS test shortly after the event in question, and Deitch did testify that Tan pricked her finger with the contaminated syringe. But the photographer had lied and Deitch was no better as a witness. Tan may have gotten HIV tested for the elite dating service in which she was enrolled. And as for crying and ripping up photos of herself and Boland, Tan might not have done it with malice, but as an illustration of her love. As to their intentions, shrugged Judge Ritter, they're difficult to discern. This was not a normal relationship.

The plot is even more tangled than the courtroom drama. There is a New Zealand tycoon, a former dean of business, from a prominent Canadian family. He was charged with conspiracy and said to have splashed Boland's face with sulfuric acid (the charges have since been stayed). And there was Tan's Fairy Godfather, an investment firm exec, who feared his own disgrace. Both had sex with Tan and lavished her with wealth. There was also some false accusation concerning Boland and drug-trafficking. But except for her threat against Jeanette Kunkel, Tan was acquitted of all charges. The former model smiled as friends and relatives rushed to her in congratulations.

No one will ever know if Tan infected Boland or not. He failed to prove that she was the source of his infection. In more general terms, Tan was acquitted because the vagaries of their lifestyle put them outside the scope of judicial assessment. As the judge said, theirs was not a normal relationship. Dalton (1993, 250) points out that a fundamental weakness of intentional HIV transmission trials is that they assume there is a common reference, that judges, juries, and defendants share a way of viewing the world such that they can assess the relevance of abstract concepts like indifference and maliciousness in the lives of those in question. He warns that more often than not, judges and juries lack a common set of values and concerns. As a result, they tend to make biased and arbitrary decisions that weigh most heavily on poor and powerless defendants (Aiken and Musheno 1994).

The strongest contrast between the Tan and the Fitzsimmons-Hebert cases is class, in both senses of the word. Tan's cool and calculating demeanor (at least as it is portrayed in the press) leads you to believe that she might, after all, have committed the perfect crime. Heinous though murder by injection is, the press fed nicely on the story. They were comfortable with the participants' celebrity. It tied nicely into the lowest common denominator of classic plots: rich woman/scorned woman. The suicide murders of unknown and ugly Fitzsimmons and Hebert (mug shots accompany their story), rise in public consciousness for a horrible irrepressible moment before sliding into oblivion. But the cases have one thing in common: They are both out of the ordinary.

Crimes of violence tend to be perceived as ordinary when the action follows certain expected scenarios or paradigms (Miller 1993). Needle attacks in defined contexts like robberies fit into ready-made categories. Take the case of HIV-infected Sylvie Trudeau, who stabbed Georgette Plouffe in Montreal after Plouffe refused to supply her with drugs. Trudeau was sentenced to thirty months in prison on charges of uttering death threats and aggravated assault. It is not known if the needle used was indeed infected or if Plouffe seroconverted as a result (Guillot Hurtubise 1996). Because Trudeau's act fits easily into traditional notions about crimes of violence, the application of criminal law makes sense.

Most crime is mundane. You'd never know it from the media, which depend on typification, exaggeration, drama, randomness, and irrationality to hold audience attention (Best 1991). So we are unlikely to read about all the people who use dirty needles because the police have the power to arrest them if they are carrying a clean one; nor are we likely to read about the widespread damage this type of police action does to public health. The media is a bottom feeder, skipping past the mundane, quick to pick up and dramatize themes from the political unconscious. When no one could figure out why Andrew Cunanan killed five men and then himself, including celebrity designer Versace, the media circulated a theory that he was motivated by "AIDS rage." When his corpse turned out to be HIV-negative, it "deepened the mystery" (Associated Press 1997). Yes, AIDS rage would have explained everything.

12 / Everything I Have Is Yours

Paranoid Mirror

In *Love in Taba,* a film shown on Cairo television in 1992, three Egyptian men are seduced by Western women at a resort town. The women left them notes saying: "Welcome to the world of AIDS." You may have heard variants. In the first I heard, the note was written in lipstick (or shaving cream?) on the bathroom mirror. The story encodes differential reactions to the epidemic; it's never just about AIDS (Fine 1992; Goldstein 1992). The story's structure is accommodating. Compare the Egyptian film script with a personal experience narrative that my friend's friend told him about how she was coming home from a great vacation on a Caribbean isle. She was at the airport when she received a box from the man she'd been pleasurin' with. The box had a little coffin inside with a message that said . . . well, you know the rest.[1]

This story works like a rumor, it crosses up myth and reality as it circulates, giving form and presence to the suppressed paranoia of those who continue to have casual sex.[2] Besides starring in the Egyptian film, the story has appeared on at least one talk show.[3] It's about as global as rumors get these days.

Television is famous for exaggeration, so I was surprised to find that the U.S. industry did not magnify extreme cases like those of Fitzsimmons-Hebert and Tan (Chapter 11). As far as I could tell from my sample, the more common televised portrayals of the problem of intentional HIV transmission concentrate on the "worried well," the heteros who have heard of AIDS as a danger spreading secretly in the bodies of dates and spouses. In its never-ending reach for market share, television has created a mythical domain that addresses the concerns of what I have come to recognize as the anxious norm. The anxious norm is an emotional state characteristic of heteros who, for one reason or another, do not assume responsibility for safe sex and hence approach their sexual pleasures with a mixture of anticipation and fear. (I define it as characteristically hetero not because people who identify as gays, lesbians, bisexuals, or transgendered don't feel this type of anxiety, but because they don't fit squarely into the television market sense of norm.)

This chapter focuses on the subject of intentional HIV transmission among heteros by featuring the stories of five seropositive characters located at different sites along the fact-fiction continuum. The first story, "Radio Witch," blurs the boundary between fact and fiction as it crosses into radio, print, and television. Patching together shreds of evidence that the story's HIV-positive antihero actually exists and that she is carrying out her threat to infect others is a central concern in all venues. The story's circulation produces an uncertainty that resonates with the anxious norm. Despite its insubstantiality, the antihero's voice is powerful enough to call out a real officer of the law.

Radio Witch at the Dating Game

> *She's sleeping with everybody she can. She is quite literally a walking time bomb that is . . . we can assume, assassinating every bed partner that she can. . . . I'm gonna hide everybody I know in the basement.*
>
> —Phil Donahue, December 27, 1991

Talk shows are the oldest and most durable of TV genres, long considered a spectacle of forced exaggerations and more recently an opening for alternative discourses (Carpignano et al. 1993). Multiple

CRIME

points of view are the basis for its structure. Narrators of personal experience provide content and authenticity. Experts present a rational overlay, usually in the form of a logical divide that fails to decrease anxiety, and in its failure, worsens it.

In the quote above, Donahue (1991) was talking about a voice dubbed "C. J." on his TV talk show. She'd been calling a disc jockey on a Dallas radio show to tell people she had AIDS, that some man gave her AIDS, and she was going to get revenge by having unsafe sex with any man who gets weak behind a pretty body and by not disclosing her HIV-status. (She is not unlike [ex?-] prostitute Deborah Johnson of Lexington, except that C. J. spoke out long before she ever got caught, *if* she ever got caught.) Donahue read a letter that had been published in *Ebony* three months earlier:

> I have AIDS. No one knows it. I go to clubs more now so I
> can meet new men. I feel that I am a beautiful person and
> I couldn't believe I got it. I sleep with four different men a
> week, sometimes more. I've slept with 48 men so far, some
> of them married. I feel if I have to die of a horrible disease, I
> won't go alone. I know I'm not right in what I am doing. Can
> you tell me what's wrong with me? Why don't I feel guilty?
>
> — *C. J.*
> *Dallas, Texas*

C. J. may have been a hoax (someone trying to scare everybody into safer sex perhaps), but the deejay said that he met her once. One night two Decembers back, when he was working a station promotion called Dating Game, she walked up to him. He'd gotten a letter just like the one she wrote to *Ebony*. She told the deejay that she was C. J. and that she was about to start her mission. He never saw her again. This is the one and only moment that her voice and body came together in public space-time.

C. J.'s story was just one example of people who intentionally spread the AIDS virus presented on Donahue's 1991 show. A taste of her shadowy case opens the show, followed by other people whose images accompanied their bodies, who by example and explanation move the paranoid impulse inherent in her story forward from quasi-fiction to reality. Donahue repeats the historical progression of the U.S. epidemic, beginning his ("not an") inquisition with two gay men. There was Victor, who does not inform sexual partners that he has AIDS but who has always engaged in "safer" ("nothing's perfect") sex since he was informed of his diagnosis in 1982. There was Michael Elmer, whose first love waited ten months to inform him that he'd tested positive, a trauma that precipitated a brief low period during which he engaged in prostitution. With Donahue's prodding, Elmer admitted that he didn't always use condoms with clients, many of whom (like his first love) also had sex with women. By this point, Donahue had successfully pushed the narrative impulse toward the fear, communicated by public health experts in the late 1980s, that HIV would move out of the gay male and injecting drug user networks into the "general population" (Cook and Colby 1992). Once at the anxious gay-hetero boundary, he brought in C. J. via the deejay from Dallas. She was followed by one Patrick Archer, a gay man from the (yes, AIDS is everywhere) Midwest, whose lover, looking tearfully out into some ocean, told him that he had lied when he had said that he was HIV-negative, a lie that he apparently had repeated to five other people, one of whom was suing. Archer was infected, although he wasn't the one who caused his former lover to be extradited in hand-cuffs from New York to Michigan. This drama, Donahue pointed out, is being played out between hetero couples as well as gay couples. Before opening the show to the audience, he addressed Barbara Emes, who'd had condomless sex with four or five sexual partners without disclosing her HIV-positive serostatus, probably because she was in denial, afraid of being rejected by her lovers, or afraid of losing her job as a hospice nurse (alibi variants arose throughout the interview).

Donahue worked toward maximal audience arousal, reinforcing

his inquisitorial format by setting the tone for audience participation: "There is ongoing widespread, ubiquitous, frequent unsafe sex between straight and gay intimate partners." (He gave no reference.) After a discussion, mostly about responsibility and blame, the eighteenth audience member had the final say: "I would hope that after this show airs that the Dallas police would make more of an effort to find this C. J." The deejay from Dallas agreed.

C. J. talked to the deejay on September 3, 1991. Donahue taped the show sometime between then and December 27, when the show aired. Sometime between these dates the Dallas police let Donahue know that they had learned that C. J. was a double hoax, a fifteen-year-old girl and a twenty-nine-year-old man. Donahue explained this in his introduction, calling the two individuals phone terrorists.

Almost two years later, on October 18, 1993, a real live assistant district attorney from Dallas showed up on the TV show *Justice Files* looking for C. J. He wanted to prosecute her under Texas' new law making it a felony to intentionally spread HIV.

C. J. freaked a lot of people out, especially guys in Dallas. Like Madonna gone psycho, she took control of her own myth, but C. J. used it to torture people, not entertain them. No crime-victim narrative for her; she was going to take control of the situation. Nor did she go for the "prisoner repents" genre, like Deborah Johnson's story about how she *used to* want to give her clients HIV but now she wants to educate them. C. J. seized the day. She radioed out an angry cry of death all across that big Texas sky. And, in the end (I imagine), she will be vanquished only by the virus, if she exists.

The public's fear of "AIDS rage" has been mobilized in group political action as well, attempting to replace fear as motivator where appeals to sense and compassion fail. As Elinor Burkett (1995, 313) recounts: the PWA Army distributed fliers in a meeting of federally funded AIDS researchers in 1994. The fliers announced in bold print, "You've fucked US long enough—Now WE'RE gonna fuck you and your sons and your daughters. . . . The PWA Army is a group of people with AIDS and HIV who are willing to sacrifice their lives to save the lives of current and future PWA's. Beginning October 1, 1994, we will EACH infect at least two HIV-negative people per day if the following demand is not met."

The PWA Army demanded a cabinet-level AIDS coordinator. The demand seems out of proportion with their threat, even if they never intended to realize their words in action. They took control of the paranoid myths in which they have figured, and there must be some satisfaction in that. But mining the political unconscious for political strategy is an unpredictable game, and they're not the only ones playing. How many people will distinguish carefully between this political action and the *completely unfounded* Christian evangelical novelists' fiction that gay activists throw HIV-positive blood on their enemies and pressure the government to use defenseless fetuses for HIV research (Colson and Vaughn 1995, cited in Minkowitz 1996)?

Come to think of it, if C. J.'s real, she might be one of those people writing "Welcome to the world of AIDS" on guys' mirrors.

Anthropomorphizing the Virus

Without the stability and coherence of traditional culture, myth in contemporary societies has less of a chance than ever of helping people resolve social contradiction. Nonetheless, two fictional TV dramas that deal with the subject of intentional HIV transmission do aspire to that function. At least they come closer to resolving contradiction and calming fear than talk shows like Donahue's, which entertain by inciting panic. The functional difference in the two genres seems to be fairly independent of content. Their function, in terms of affect on public consciousness, seems to be determined by narrative structure. The talk shows induce uncontrolled plots, creating a subject at loose ends. Fictional drama presents a more coherent plot, centered around a moral contradiction that moves toward resolution as the narrative progresses. Given the quickness of TV drama and its lack of character development, the stories tend to objectify and mythify positions and solutions. They're a bit too slick to take to heart.

The two detective dramas I include here work toward different kinds of closure, style and perspective, although both share a simple four-part plot structure: (1) setup (meet characters, sketch situation); (2) investigation (learn telling details about characters; note that *NYPD Blue* divides this part into two scenes); (3) confrontation; and (4) resolution.

NYPD Blue is a fast-paced television police drama composed of three or four fictional subplots per episode, the camera veering artistically between them. Subplots are punctuated every ten minutes or so by a signature montage of the show's star cops crossing the city streets to a New York subway drum beat, the signature montage sandwiching a string of commercials. About five years after C. J. told the deejay she was going to start her mission in Dallas, and after a host of intentional HIV transmission cases came through U.S. criminal courts and military tribunals, *NYPD Blue* ran an intentional HIV transmission subplot.[4]

Scene 1:

Beautiful young woman #1 in bed with her stricken mother at her side. Mother tells police detectives that she wishes the man who infected her daughter with HIV were dead, that shooting him down would be too good for him. But without proof that the man had been tested and informed that he himself was HIV-positive, the police say, they cannot charge him with reckless disregard. They are not currently pursuing any cases in this area of endangerment.

ads and narrative fragments

• • • • • from other subplot(s) • • • • •

Scene 2:

As coincidence would have it, the man in question gets picked up on a minor charge. He already had drug offenses on record. A routine drug war alibi creates an opening for the police detectives to poke around.[5]

ads and narrative fragments
• • • • • from other subplot(s) • • • • •

Scene 3:

Detectives find sex partner #2, a healthy-looking HIV-positive woman. She already knows how and why #1 was infected and that she is dying, and she has been trying to warn sex partner #3. Sex partner #2 said the man in question was crazy and into selling drugs. When once she asked him about AIDS, he said, "Do I look like I have AIDS? I've never been sick, why should I be tested?"

ads and narrative fragments
• • • • • from other subplot(s) • • • • •

Scene 4:

Detectives find sex partner #3. She says she met the handsome guy in a gym where he worked as a trainer. The cops gently tried to break the news about the other two women, suggesting that she get tested. [The test and her reaction to the news that she is positive happens off-screen.]

We are looking (from the perspective of the police) at the body of the infector shot dead in the street. Sex partner #3 is crying on the neighboring stoop. "That's what he deserved," she said. The gun was in her purse. The detectives arrest her and offer her a plea. The lawyer says the plea will never go to sentence. The woman cop says, "She already got her sentence."

The TV camera lends its audience cops' eyes: corporate networks define the scope of social problems for the masses. Note that the police detectives don't actually prevent anything from happening. The police seem like they're in the flow, almost as unsure as anybody else encountering this type of situation for the first time. But it's their warning that induces sex partner # 3 to get tested, the results of which trigger murder. (Number 3 could have benefited from pre- and post-test counseling.) The closing line, when the woman cop says, "She's already got her sentence," echoes the voice of the real Terry Fitzsimmons, the Canadian psycho who injected his crime partner's tainted blood as his own self-delivered capital punishment (Chapter 9). In fictional television drama the speaker is a compassionate cop talking about a victim (sex partner # 3) who takes justice into her own hands, but the thought is the same: AIDS is a death sentence that can be inflicted at will. The unspoken implication of this *NYPD Blue* episode is that we don't have enough laws to let the cops do it right, or, although this type of crime is heinous, it is too slippery to define and control. The first implication harbors a threat; that is, if we don't give the state power to control this type of behavior, citizens will take things into their own hands (echoing the real case of Deborah Johnson who, in lieu of a waived death sentenced for LaFonda Fay Foster, tried to kill her co-inmate with HIV-infected blood [Chapter 9]).

NYPD Blue exploits an old motif (three maidens give themselves to a man who is not what he seems) to present a new crime (intentional HIV transmission). The actor's bad man's charm is disturbing because it is not unlike the kind of man with whom many women viewers might consider having sex. The Terry Fitzsimmonses of the world may be easier for our imaginations to cope with. At least they're up front and quick about their murderous intentions and they're far too grotesque to have ever been invited into our sexual fantasies. Fitzsimmons types rear up from the political unconscious only to sink deeper. It's the normal, good-looking ones pleasure-seeking women ought to worry about. I'm sure Phil Donahue would agree.

Television scriptwriters sometimes set their writing to work against stereotypes. Rather than trying to invent and communicate in a new language, they usually set up the same old scenario, reversing audience expectations regarding a character in a particular role or an outcome. On May 2, 1996, a British detective show shown on U.S. public television's *Mystery* series set up an intentional HIV transmission scenario, reversing the usual cops-eye view in the end by transforming the evil infector into a fellow sufferer. An hour-long drama uninterrupted by commercial breaks or subplots, the narrative was told from the perspective of Ellie, private eye in a two-woman team called Chandler and Company. This rough plot summary omits scenes about Ellie's personal life:

Scene 1:

An Anglican priest's daughter dies of AIDS while at college. He hires Ellie to find out which college boy infected her.

Scene 2:

Ellie goes to the college and talks to people who knew her. She finds the daughter's diary in her room and learns of her burgeoning sexual passion. She also learns the boy is a man.

Scene 3:

Ellie finds the man in the college video equipment room. She enters the room more or less ready to confront a suspect, but instead, finds a doomed, grief-stricken man. He tells her that he was an ex-drug injector who must have gotten infected in his youth. He and the daughter had always used condoms, but there was one time when she didn't want to; "It was about intimacy," the daughter had said. The woman detective and the man with AIDS hug and cry.

Scene 4:

The last scene takes place outside on one of those college greenswards in a venerable stone quadrangle with long, wide paths. The daughter's lover-infector walks up to the priest after his daughter's funeral service and the priest rejects his handshake. But in a swiftly following redemptive moment the priest calls out to the infected man and they hug as fellow sufferers.

The Chandler and Company drama blurs the binary image of innocent maiden – evil male infector, confusing the mythic assignment of blame. Despite our tendency to want to despise the source of HIV in our loved ones' lives, the well-meaning public TV writers and producers tell us, we should be able to evolve to the point where we recognize our common humanity (and potential victimhood).

Would that we could leave it at that. . . . And maybe we could, except that some HIV-infected people don't stop after they've infected one other person. As in the *NYPD Blue* version, it is the serial nature of the act that forces public confrontation.

The next story is based on a real case. The talk show incoherence and dramatic fiction's simplicity disappear. We are left instead with a depressing list of unromantic sexual details drained of all traces of affection.

> *MURDER HAS ITS SEXUAL SIDE*
> —*Jenny Holzer, Truisms, 1983*
> (excerpt from a circulating electronic string)

A Small Time Con from Oregon

Timothy Hinkhouse's only television appearance was a prosecutor's footnote on *Justice Files*.[6] The show's title was "Love and Death." The lead-in quote was "He knew he had the HIV virus. But he hid it from the women who loved him." The prime perp, one Alberto Gonzalez, allegedly infected two women (one of whom had died of AIDS) and raped a seventeen-year-old girl. He was convicted on one charge of attempted murder in 1992 and sentenced to nine and a half years in prison.

In terms of audience draw, the Hinkhouse case was undistinguished. As far as I can tell, there was a complete lack of big-time media interest in him, despite the multiplicity of his victims and the relative novelty of associating HIV infection with crime. His case is not an outtake because it is extreme or bizarre like the Fitzsimmons-Hebert and Tan cases, but quite the opposite: It's depressingly mundane. Hinkhouse, unfortunately, might not be doing something that out of the ordinary. He got caught only because he was an offender already under the supervision of the criminal justice system. In that sense, his case is most similar to those of prostitutes like Deborah Johnson. New forms of intervention, like criminal prosecution for intentional HIV transmission, are focused more intensively on those who are already under police surveillance.

The court of appeals opinion pertaining to the Hinkhouse case scrolled across the screen in the Lexis survey of intentional HIV transmission. The opinion was written by Judge Landau of the Court of Appeals of Oregon on March 6, 1996; I retell the story from the court transcript.[7]

In summary: Hinkhouse was convicted of ten counts of attempted murder and ten counts of attempted assault, based on his conduct of engaging in unprotected sexual intercourse with a number of victims without disclosing his medical condition. On appeal, he argued that the convictions must be set aside, because the evidence was insufficient to establish that he intended to cause the death of, or serious physical injury to, any of his several victims. The judges agreed with the state that the evidence was sufficient to support the convictions and affirmed the circuit court judge's decision.

Following Landau's published opinion, the facts of the case are told in the light most favorable to the state (and paraphrased here):

Sex partner #1:
■   Hinkhouse knew he was HIV-positive in 1989 when he had sex with fifteen-year-old P. B. He moved to California, but then came back, continuing the sexual relationship. He would not use condoms, didn't

like them, he said. They never talked about AIDS. He left town again in July 1990 and mentioned that she might want to get a test. By August she was officially positive. A few months later he called and they met. He asked her if she'd been tested. "Well, you know my status because you gave it to me," she said. He brushed her comment off.

In November of 1990, Hinkhouse told his probation officer that he was HIV-positive, and the officer immediately explained the seriousness of the disease, how it was transmitted, why he should use condoms, and that it would be like killing someone if he passed the virus on to someone else. This discussion was repeated during the next few months, and the officer cautioned him again once on the phone: "If you infect one, that is murder." Hinkhouse said he understood and agreed to take precautions. This went on into 1992, when Hinkhouse was taken into custody again for a probation violation. Hinkhouse told the officer that he would "cease and desist from any kind of sexual activity." But not only did he continue to engage in sex with a number of women, he was heard bragging about his prowess and lack of concern for exposing them. When released, he signed a probation agreement that committed him to abstaining from unsupervised contact with women without express permission from his probation officer. In 1993, he had several sexual relationships without notifying the probation officer. In each case, he refused to use a condom during sex and failed to disclose his HIV status.

Sex partner # 2:
■   In May of 1993, he began having sex with P. D. He never used a condom nor said anything about HIV.

Sex partner # 3:
■   In June of 1993, he began having sex with L. K. She demanded that he use a condom, and for three or four weeks he did. One time he promised but didn't, in spite of her protests. They had a long talk about

safe sex, he told her how he'd just ended a long-term relationship, how he'd not engaged in any risky behavior since then, and how he'd recently tested negative for HIV. L. K. and Hinkhouse resumed having sex. He kept skipping the condoms. When she expressed concern, he told her there was no need, if either of them had HIV, the other was already exposed. He said he would get tested, but didn't follow through. There was a brief hiatus before L. K. took up with him again. He became rough, making her bleed when they had intercourse. When she complained, he was casual, even proud. He attempted to enter her anally several times, even though she was dead set against it. He could be gentle, L. K. said, but he became rough, rude, mean, spiteful, hurtful. She ended the relationship that August.

Sex partner # 4

■   By September Hinkhouse began having sex with R. L. She suggested he buy condoms. He told her that he didn't believe in them. She said he could have HIV. He said, "I don't . . . have it, and whoever is telling you is lying."

Sex partner # 5

■   Around the same time Hinkhouse began seeing R. L. (# 4), he started a relationship with M. S. (# 5). With M. S. it was romantic. Hinkhouse hoped that he and M. S. would marry one day. He told M. S. that he was HIV-positive and always used condoms with her.

Three experts testified: The doctor explained the dynamics of transmission, pointing out the increased risk of violent and anal sex, explaining that a person may be infected after a single exposure. The psychologist testified that Hinkhouse was just acting out sexually, and his reported 1991 threat that he would "go out and spread" HIV could not be given much credence. The man, he said, had attention deficit disorder (a childhood disease) and simply did not consider the consequences of his acts. The state's expert agreed with the psychologist insofar as attention deficit disorder, adding borderline personality disorder and antisocial behavior to the diagnosis. He reminded the judge that when his probation officer warned him against infecting other people, Hinkhouse said that "he was going to do whatever he wanted, whenever he wanted." Hinkhouse used condoms with the one woman for whom he expressed genuine romantic interest, but declined to use them with any of the others. Hinkhouse reportedly had a conversation with another former lover and told her that if he were HIV-positive, he would spread the virus to other people. In the state's expert's opinion, Hinkhouse showed a pattern of systematically recruiting and exploiting multiple partners over time. His behavior showed intentional, deliberate conduct. There was no evidence to suggest that Hinkhouse was merely being impulsive or careless. Three judges agreed.

Hinkhouse was on a search-and-destroy mission. And unlike the paranoid mirror's threatening scribbler or C. J. the Radio Witch, we know Hinkhouse is real. Except for the pathological diagnoses of the psychologist and state's expert, which seem distant from the knot of ethical dilemmas at issue, we don't know what Hinkhouse was thinking. His voice is silenced in the transcript.

Nevertheless, the court testimony of five women raises questions about the meaning of consensual in the phrase "consensual sex." Why didn't the women insist on using condoms? Was it their own sexual desires that made them susceptible to Hinkhouse's pressure? The ideal presumes that each individual has a more or less equal access to AIDS education; that understanding of HIV transmission is linked directly to risk reduction behavior; that risk reduction behavior proceeds in a consistent fashion whether or not one knows the serostatus of one's sexual partner; and finally, that everyone has an equal ability to determine the level of their own risk in a sexual relationship. While the ideal may be the best institutional stance to take when considering the pandemic's population-level impact, it clearly sacrifices certain individuals and groups who are at a disadvantage.

There has been some research, mostly on gay and bisexual men, focusing on the role of self-disclosure of positive HIV serostatus in sexual decision making. Data show that the majority of seropositive men tell their primary partners about their HIV infection (69 to 98 percent), but when more casual secondary partners are taken into account, rates of self-disclosure are much lower (7 to 47 percent) (see review in Sobo 1995, 57–60). (It was the reported difference between the way Hinkhouse treated the woman he cared about and the way he treated his previous sex partners that damned him in the eyes of the court.) In a study of 223 HIV-positive homosexual, heterosexual, and bisexual men participating in substance abuse or AIDS prevention programs, 61 men (26 percent) characterized as sexually compulsive had a history of unprotected anal, vaginal, and oral sex with multiple partners. The 61 men placed hundreds of sex partners at risk of infection in a relatively short period of time, leading researchers to call for prevention strategies for people who know they are infected and who have difficulty protecting their sexual partners (Kalichman et al. 1997). The problem does not just reside in nondisclosure, however, because couples who *know,* whether hetero or homosexual, that one of them can infect the other (discordant couples) continue to engage in high-risk practices (Padian 1990). In any case, what data there are suggest that Hinkhouse and his five sex partners are not unique.

The majority of defendants in intentional HIV transmission court cases between 1986 and 1996 involve men charged with infecting women with whom they are having casual sex.[8] The Hinkhouse case is one of seventeen U.S. cases that I found for this period in which HIV-related criminal charges were brought against adults involved in consensual sexual relations. Of these, all the defendants but three were heterosexual men. The other three charged were women, but one was judged mentally incompetent to stand trial, and one claims to have been drunk and raped during the incident in question.[9]

In Canada, the Ssenyonga case brought the shortcomings of the public health counseling system into sharp relief. Charles Ssenyonga

CRIME

was a charming and well-educated man who came to Canada to study in 1983 after escaping war in his native Uganda, an epicenter of the AIDS pandemic. He came to the attention of a family doctor in Toronto a few years later, when she diagnosed three women as being HIV-positive. All identified Ssenyonga as their most recent sexual contact. Although warned repeatedly by public health officials, and under court order to refrain from certain unprotected activities, Ssenyonga allegedly continued to infect women. He was eventually charged with criminal negligence causing bodily harm, administering a noxious thing, and common nuisance. He died before conviction (Calwood 1995). There are at least seven Canadian cases to date in which criminal charges were mounted against adults engaged in consensual sex; only one of these was a woman (Elliot 1997, Appendix B, 1–17).

As the court waded through, and imposed order on, the wayward complexity of Hinkhouse's recent past, the mundane intimacies of violence in the sexual mode do not lead to agreement. The experts chosen to inform the court's judgment are scanty and haphazard. They reduce the complexities of social reality to pathological motive and the complexities of epidemiology to the Achilles' heel of science: while science can say that the chances of HIV transmission occurring in a single sex act is improbable, it cannot say that it is impossible.[10]

However, there is no doubt that HIV can be used as a weapon. Once framed in this way, the problem requires legal solution. To reach that solution in the Hinkhouse case, the appeals process resembles a variant on the basic four-part plot structure used in detective fiction: the setup (the court's case summary) is followed by an investigation (testimony of victims); confrontation (referring back to earlier confrontations between probation officer and Hinkhouse); and resolution (denial of appeal). But unlike the mythic resolutions posed by detective fiction (have a victim shoot the perp before he gets to court or transform the perp in question back into an innocent victim), even ten convictions of attempted murder cannot bring closure. At least four women had unprotected sex with Hinkhouse and one is confirmed infected. Meanwhile, Hinkhouse faces a slow, mean prison death. Reality is messy. There are no ready-made answers in the domains of law, popular culture, or public health. The central dilemma is the irresolvability of defining HIV infection as a "crime."

Hinkhouse is an easy mark: a repeated probation violator with a big mouth, a paper trail documenting his test results and AIDS education, five witnesses ready to testify against him, and reason to lock him up. The next story is about a man whose deeds are not very different from Hinkhouse's, but whose celebrity affords him special protection. He died before he went to court and Morley Safer of *60 Minutes* did a postmortem.

But first, a final note of wishful, not terribly unrealistic thinking: Given recent history, it seems inevitable that states will continue to find ways of prosecuting individuals who intentionally transmit HIV or who knowingly have unprotected sex without disclosing a positive HIV serostatus. In order to assure that new forms of prosecution work are governed by principles of fairness and equality according to the aims of public health and civil rights, it is crucial that criminal law is used only as a last resort. The establishment of adequate treatment programs and social welfare supports for HIV-positive persons and a coherent and enforceable set of antidiscrimination laws should precede any further moves toward criminalization.

The Hero

The narrative structure of magazine news shows like *60 Minutes* seems to fall somewhere between talk shows and fiction. They deal with real cases that incite the anxious norm. They are more tightly produced than talk shows and project a greater moral authority than either talk shows or fiction, characteristics that tend to add to their mythifying power. In the intentional HIV transmission story that follows, plot structure reproduces fictional narrative through the setup,

investigation, and confrontation. Like the talk show, the news magazine segment rests in contradiction rather than resolution.

"ATHLETES: THE WOMEN IN THEIR LIVES," reads the
graphic backdrop of Morley Safer's *60 Minutes* piece on November 10, 1996, in which he presents a commercially uninterrupted segment on the question of intentional HIV transmission from the perspective of Lagena Lookabill Greene, victim of famous race car driver
Tim Richmond. Although based on reported fact, and presented in a
much more orderly fashion than the fictional *NYPD Blue* segment,
60 Minutes contributes to the solidification of public thinking about
this type of crime around its majority stereotype: white, hetero relationships in which femininity is tied to victimhood. My retelling is
based on the *60 Minutes* transcript and a column from the *Winnipeg
Sun* (CBS News 1996; Associated Press 1996):

■   Richmond told no one of his infection, though he learned of it in
1986. He was a race car hero, flamboyant on and off the track. Fans in
the stands and money in the bank, was what the promoters thought.

Just what racing needed, fast-driving, on the edge. Richmond didn't
need no publicist, had no use for advertisers, 'cause the female fans
they flocked. He was a good-looking guy, dashing in fact with a taste
for promiscuity. Women's betting jumped 25 percent when he raced
at the track. Addicted to competition, was what he said about himself.

Pit lizards, they called them, the motor racing groupies. Lookabill
wasn't part of that scene. Lookabill was a beauty queen who met Richmond at the Charlotte Motor Speedway. She supposed he was in-
trigued by her, because she didn't throw herself at him. They had a
brief encounter that went nowhere at first.

Lookabill was an A student at the University of North Carolina.
She moved to L.A. after graduation, and in movies and TV met modest
success. She did see Richmond from time to time, but she thought it
was pure friendship. She had a boyfriend, Danny Greene, whom she

later married. But in 1986, they had parted ways. And Lookabill returned to Charlotte.

She had a part in a racing car movie, but emotionally was unsteady. After two marriage proposals and six years of pursuit, Richmond made his move. Lookabill thought he was ready to settle down.

She agreed to join him on a publicity trip, a harmless one day in New York. They got a hotel room and he proposed, and that time she accepted. And in that room they did have unprotected sex. She thought they'd be married soon. They were to have Thanksgiving in L.A., but he never showed up or called. Richmond dropped totally out of sight. Lookabill never saw him again.

Some time later she began receiving calls, reporters checking rumors that Richmond had AIDS. Richmond even went on CBS Sports to tell the world it was only a touch of pneumonia, triggered by a bit of Asian flu. Lookabill had herself tested and found out she was HIV-positive.

When Richmond made a brief comeback, his fans idolized him for overcoming adversity. Lookabill stayed silent until Tim Richmond died. She'd envisioned the glaring faces of 180,000 fans who would hate her for telling the truth about their beloved macho man.

It's not clear what Richmond knew and when he knew it, whether it was before or after Lookabill's night in New York. She does believe that he had AIDS that night and she does accept some responsibility, after all, she was not raped. But she cannot really fathom how another human being could knowingly expose her to this virus.

The courage that he showed around the celebrity track was not enough to save him from hurting Lookabill. Richmond never did concede to AIDS even up until his death. So he didn't have to face the AP headline: "Race With Death *Driver infects dozens of women.*" Lookabill knows at least two other women who have said they tested positive and one woman who has died as a result of sex with Richmond. The deceased one's grandmother came on TV and thought out loud about

CRIME

the many women who stay quiet. She figures they haven't come forward to tell the world what Richmond did because they're afraid the world would see them as villains or tramps. In some circles, Richmond is still revered and was recently inducted into the Eastern Motor Sports Hall of Fame.

This is much like the story of the Regent—the fans are acting like a community with a sacred text. The sacred text requires humans, like the Regent and Tim Richmond, to perform heroic roles. These roles offer extraordinary protection, seemingly allowing heroes to overcome the greatest dangers. Belief in heroic roles thus mutes acknowledgment of AIDS. Followers become addicted to the specific states of enlightenment or pleasure induced in their group's connection. The Buddhists were addicted to the notion that the Regent was the closest thing to enlightenment this side of the Buddha. Richmond's racing fans were addicted to the excitement and speed of spectatorship, gambling, and masculine prowess.

But sports is supposed to be a family values kind of thing, and sports heroes have to be virtuous sex maniacs, or the formula won't work (Sally Jenkins on *60 Minutes*, CBS News 1996, 21). Tim Richmond telling his fans that he has AIDS is telling them that their most thrilling fantasies are diseased. No one wants to face this. Unwilling to endure public disappointment, Richmond sacrificed the women who helped create his heroic aura. Though Thomas Rich, the Regent, may have stood awfully close to enlightenment and Tim Richmond, the driver, may have been a national hero, in the end neither man may have been that different from unknowns like Tim Hinkhouse, Deborah Johnson, or (if she exists) C. J., the Radio Witch: None of them could face the cosmic fact of their own insignificance, and all were willing to impose their awful fate on anyone who came within their sexual sphere. Without any consciousness at all, HIV has the capacity to move in through just this kind of cultural opening.

Told from the victim's perspective, this story gives insight into the process of public recognition that transforms unprotected sex from "risky behavior" into "crime." Lookabill knew that she was injured by Richmond, and she also knew that she willingly had unprotected sex with him. She was not sure whether or not a social paradigm existed to confirm her sense of injury; in other words, she didn't know whether people who had been harmed as she had even had a right to complain. Given Richmond's hero status, Lookabill said that she feared she would be ridiculed or ignored and waited for his death to advance her claim. As Miller (1993, 58–59) argues, it is often not the victim who has the power to define the nature of a violent event in public discourse, but the observer. It is Morley Safer, *60 Minutes* commentator and personality, who has the authority and power to socialize Lookabill's claim. Devoured by the communication network's agents and machines, a brave Lookabill, weakened and in bed, becomes a material-semiotic node actively shaping the form that popular and legal judgment assumes (cf. Haraway 1991, 208). She was still beautiful.

Forces at Play

The uneven process in which intentional HIV transmission becomes recognized as a crime and punished moves through various semi-autonomous institutional domains. When they are not downright contentious, professionals in different domains tend to talk past each other. The court bucks the accepted public health mantra that individuals must take responsibility for themselves, focusing on controlling those in the system with the force of law. The media focus on celebrity and the anxious norm. Publicly framing and magnifying reckless and malicious individuals, the media give anthropomorphic form to viral fears. This process cannot be pushed aside as merely paranoid or persecutory fantasy, although it certainly is that.

There is a string of truisms that tend to orient AIDS researchers and activists against all moves toward criminalization. My take on

CRIME

them is the following: It is impossible for the state to distinguish between fraudulent patterns of sexual risk causing serial infection and other justifiable causes of serial infection (such as lack of control over temporary anger, denial, fear of abuse). The state's incapacity to distinguish among causes may result in the criminalization of simple risk taking (Field and Sullivan 1987). The distinction may be possible to establish in some cases, but given systemic biases and prejudices against those who are, or are perceived to be, poor, deviant, or nonwhite, laws based on such distinctions will not be enforced equally and fairly. If such distinctions can be established and applied fairly, they will nevertheless undermine the trust in public health professionals, their blood tests, and their advice, resulting in a relative increase in the overall number of HIV infections. It is safer not to expand the scope of state intrusion into private life. As Justice Thurgood Marshall (cited in Zink 1992) wrote in his dissenting opinion in *Skinner v. Railway Executive Association,* the case in which the U.S. Supreme Court upheld drug and alcohol testing of railroad employees, "When we allow fundamental freedoms to be sacrificed in the name of real or perceived exigency, we invariably come to regret it."

The list of scholar-activist truisms is cautious and well meaning; they are also ignored or trivialized by many legislators, prosecutors, and talk show hosts. Also ignored is the social reality of everyday sexual risk taking: When Donahue's gay guest mentions safe sex, he is met by the host's sarcasm; when public television conveys a message of compassionate detection, they drench it in pastel tones of utopian redemption; when the court brings in experts, testimony regarding the normal range of sexual risk taking is absent.

It is crucial to balance the stories about the Deborah Johnsons, the Tim Hinkhouses, and the Tim Richmonds with the stories of the people in "Work" and "Escape," the first two parts of the book: the Jacquis, the Boots, the Sandys, the Rosalinds, the Simones, the Maggies, the Nats, the California therapists on vacation. Networks of HIV risk are shaped by persons who experience a combination of tensions, motivations, conditions, pretensions, and desires. Whether the mode of intervention is prevention, antidiscrimination, or punishment, to be effective and fair, the agents of public health and criminal justice need to at least attempt to account for the dynamic heterogeneity of sexual risk. Maybe they'll never capture the random liveliness of carnival, but they can weigh the preponderance of evidence that social life brings to bear.

Once cases get to criminal court, it would be useful to temper paranoid abstractions with balanced epidemiological and ethnographic testimony. The epidemiological data are there, the value of testimony depends on which strategic slant the epidemiologist is hired to assume. There is little ethnographic data organized for this purpose. While there has been much ethnographic research on sexual risk taking among individuals and social networks, the scope of data collection and analysis has been determined almost entirely by the public health ideal. We understand little about the phenomenon that criminal law puts at issue: *a fraudulent pattern of sexual risk behavior that may result in serial* HIV *infections.*

More broadly, ethnographer-activists might serve as mediators between domains of public health, criminal law, and popular/mass culture. Providing translations between one professional discourse and another, grounding professional discourses in "what everybody around here knows," exposing alibis, proposing and implementing useful prevention and care strategies. To be relevant to the particular institutional intersection at issue here, ethnographer-activists must be willing to contemplate the possibility of malice in relation to disease. Consideration must extend from individual citizens to salary-paying institutions. After all, we have a massive addiction problem that is fueled by money, paranoia, and the thrills of techno-violence: *the U.S. government has a drug war habit.* Its leaders ought to take some lessons in addiction management from heroin and cocaine addicts like Rosalind (Chapter 7): "You have to have a line that you draw," she says. The U.S. government has a drug war habit and a half-hearted public health agenda is its alibi, a claim to good intentions.

It is crucial to resist feeding pretense to special knowledge and authority. The political unconscious is a reservoir from which everyone drinks, poor and rich, farmer and social scientist, talk show host and judge. There is a surprising fluidity in imagery and narrative structure in the austere and ordered discourse of the court, the statistical verities of epidemiological risk, and the paranoid deviance that the media love to hate. And as the Belizean case illustrates, imagery travels faster than the virus itself. Image, viral infection, symptomology, the availability of new treatments, and hopes for a vaccine or cure become active elements in public discourse in different temporal orders and combinations. The atmospheres of risk particular to different cultural locales are keyed into the globe-trotting wilds of the political unconscious—a mutating confabulation in which facts become distorted fantasies (for example, conspiracy theories) and fantasies become distorted facts (or an ordered universe of risk founded on deviant acts). No one is immune. Even those who struggle against its imagery find themselves addressing it in its own crazy terms. As the force of its imagery filters through the array of institutional and popular discourses active in the Americas, the political unconscious drives pandemic history.

Locked in visions of war and conquest, we steer natural selection to create a shape-shifting enemy. Seduced by visions of abstract enlightenment and embodied pleasures, we offer ourselves sublimely. HIV, the retrovirus, transcribes itself into cells and psyches. Parodying our humanity, it becomes us. We in turn must become the Trickster: Fierce pragmatism, promiscuous compassion, and a touch of mocking humor are the medicine for undoing the random power of viral mutation.

/ Notes

CHAPTER I

1. The U.S. government first began to get prevention efforts among drug injectors underway in 1987. It was six years after the Centers for Disease Control and Prevention (CDC) (1981) published findings on early isolated cases of *Pneumocystis carinii* pneumonia among young men across the United States and postulated that there might be a causative agent that was sexually transmitted.

2. The majority of scientists believe that human immunodeficiency virus (HIV) is the primary cause of AIDS. It is the most intensively studied virus in history. High-resolution microscopy shows HIV fragments (virions) to be roughly spherical and about one ten-thousandth of a millimeter across. The outer coat consists of a double layer of lipid molecules taken from membranes of surrounding human cells. The lipid coat is studded with proteins, some of human origin. The genetic material in the core of the virion is RNA, ribonucleic acid, rather than the more usual DNA, deoxyribonucleic acid. Viral RNA is transcribed into DNA once the virus enters human immune system cells. Because the RNA-to-DNA transcription process reverses the usual order of events, HIV is called a retrovirus. HIV causes profound immune dysfunction over time, indirectly causing death by means of other opportunistic diseases (Greene 1993). The composition of RNA varies among different strains and subtypes of HIV; strains vary in the nature of their infectivity and geographic distribution. Sexual transmission of HIV accounts for 75 to 85 percent of the nearly 28 million estimated HIV infections in the world (Joint United Nations Programme on HIV/AIDS 1996). For reviews that tie epidemiological models to social factors see MacQueen 1994 and Royce et al. 1997.

3. At current levels of incarceration, a black male in the United States today has a greater than one in four (28.5 percent) chance of going to prison during his lifetime, twice as likely as Hispanics (16 percent) and six times more likely than whites (4.4 percent) (U.S. Department of Justice 1997, 1).

4. See Linda Singer's analysis of the film *Fatal Attraction* for an example of how anxieties associated with the pleasure of dangerous sex play out in popular

culture (1993). For a discussion of how panic logic incites the phenomena it seeks to control, see Judith Butler's introduction to Singer, p. 9.

5. For the most recent update on needle exchange programs in the United States, see CDC (1997). A ban on allowing federal funds to be used for needle exchange programs in the United States is still in place as of fall 1997. A recent crackdown on drug-using pregnant women denies them the option of utilizing treatment programs they have only recently won the right to enter. Twenty-four U.S. states have already prosecuted (mostly black and poor) women for ingesting drugs when pregnant and for murder if their children died. The number of these prosecutions tripled between 1990 and 1992 (Breitbart, Chavkin, and Wise 1994, cited in Farmer et al. 1996). For social analysis see Roberts 1995. On criminalization of HIV-positive prostitutes see, for example, Alexander 1996.

6. George Washington University law professor David Robinson Jr. even invoked AIDS prevention as an argument in support of Georgia's law criminalizing sodomy (cited in Leonard 1993, 158).

7. As Scott and Marshall (1991, 8) point out in their discussion of the 1989 report by the Senate Subcommittee on Terrorism, Narcotics, and International Operations (known as the Kerry Report): "The history of official toleration for or complicity with drug traffickers in Central America in the 1980s suggests the inadequacy of traditional 'supply-side' or 'demand-side' drug strategies whose targets are remote from Washington. Chief among these targets have been the ethnic ghettos of America's inner cities (the demand side) and the foreign peasants who grow coca plants or opium poppies (the supply side). Experience suggests instead that one of the first targets for an effective drug strategy should be Washington itself, and specifically its own support for corrupt, drug-linked forces in the name of anticommunism."

8. More specifically, this work is an example of multisite ethnography (Marcus 1995).

9. I explore the double process of globalization: On the one hand, I trace the extension outward of one homogenized culture to its limit; on the other hand, I describe the compression of distinct local cultures brought into contact and juxtaposition through AIDS without obvious organizing principles (Featherstone 1995, 6).

10. For recent anthropological contributions to AIDS research and intervention, see, for example, Feldman 1990; Herdt and Lindenbaum 1992; Brummelhuis and Herdt 1995; Bond et al. 1997; Singer 1998.

11. The names of private individuals in Chicago have been changed to preserve anonymity.

12. AIDS law is a burgeoning field, most of which focuses on protecting the rights of those who are infected. Criminal law plays only a small part. For a comprehensive discussion, see Webber 1997; for a discussion of the criminalization debate in the United States, see, for example, Sullivan and Field 1988; Dalton 1993; for synthesis of criminal legislation in the United States, see Gostin 1996; in Canada, see Patterson 1995 and Elliot 1997.

13. I have compiled this data from a number of sources. In addition to a survey of Lexis-Nexis for this decade, I have drawn from unpublished lists of the National Conference of State Legislatures (1995) and the National Victim Center (1995). See also Hannaham's (1996) data summary in the popular gay magazine *Out*. Also note that in 1994, 27 percent of full-time prosecutors' offices serving populations of at least 500,000 people have prosecuted at least one case of "HIV exposure" (U.S. Department of Justice 1996, 3).

CHAPTER 2

1. The 1988 baseline seroprevalence among injectors from Chicago was 24 percent, with a 10 percent per person-year seroconversion rate, that is, an average of one out of ten persons became infected with HIV each year (Wiebel et al. 1990).

2. The term "toast" connotes and encompasses the corpus of African American tales from the oral tradition (for example, the Signifying Monkey, Tar Baby, the Titanic). In addition to tales per se, however, "toast" signifies jokes, legends, songs, and literary material that have been adopted from other cultures as well as from written literature (Dotson 1977, 2).

3. Tape 24, interview Aug. 15, 1988; field notes Aug. 16, 1988, pp. 14ff.

4. Field notes, Oct. 28, 1988, pp. 65–66.

5. M. Daniel Fernando (1993) writes that one might cynically conclude that AIDS researchers' reliance on bleach distribution and needle exchange is motivated by their desire to perpetuate a fundable niche for their work. If clean needles were widely accessible and decriminalized (as they are in the Netherlands), there would be little need for the kind of research and intervention programs that NIDA funds.

6. See Kane and Mason 1992 for critical analysis of NIDA-funded ethnographic research on sex partners and injecting drug users. Frankenburg (1995) provides an insightful review of the conflicts anthropologists have encountered working on interdisciplinary team projects structured according to epidemiological categories.

7. For a feminist analysis of Loki's toast, see Kane 1993.

CHAPTER 3

1. From interviews with the artist Gerald Chavanne, who was designing AIDS intervention posters for the nongovernmental organization Project Hope (Jan. 9, 1990) and Mrs. Courtney (Feb. 9, 1990), director general of Red Cross. Note that the WHO health representative chose to ignore the Belize Ministry of Health report of fifty-five AIDS cases and fifteen deaths by 1989. The first AIDS case was reported in 1986 and attributed to heterosexual transmission (Belize Ministry of Health 1990). The transmission dynamics in Belize may well turn out to be closer to that of the English-speaking Caribbean and Africa, with a fairly equal proportion of infections occurring among men and women alike, rather than to the United States, with a higher ratio of male-to-female infections. Note that, like the chapters on the Chicago project, the names of private persons in Belize have been changed to preserve anonymity.

2. For 1996–1997, Belize reported 198 AIDS cases; Mexico 29,962; Honduras 6,057; El Salvador 1,875; and Guatemala 1,787 (WHO 1997). In the six years between this most recent report and my field research, reported AIDS cases have multiplied considerably, with Belize, the country with the smallest apparent problem, reporting a seventeenfold increase in cases, and Mexico, the country with the apparent largest problem, reporting a threefold increase. Accounting for variations in population does not significantly change the range of increase. The increase in official cases is partly due to the expanded case definition of AIDS, which began to include women's gynecological symptoms in 1994 (WHO 1994).

3. In his books, Cantwell (1988, 1993), a physician, argues for the medical origin of AIDS, presenting evidence that HIV was originally spread in New York by clinical trials carried out on gay men for a Hepatitis B vaccine. See also Chapter 7, note 3.

4. Tom Curtis (1992) explores the theory that African AIDS was spread via the polio vaccine.

5. As I write this chapter I hear a *National Public Radio* report (evening news, Oct. 2, 1996) that Haitian radio station WLQY in south Florida is declaring that the AIDS epidemic is a myth, an invention by American drug companies, and that Haitians who are being treated for the disease should stop. An epidemiologist with the Dade County Health Department reports increasing problems with AIDS patient compliance as a result. The epidemiologist explains that because educational levels are not high, people base their decisions on individuals whom they trust rather than scientific information. They are distrustful of government in general, he said, due to the fact that sixteen years ago, when the epidemic first started, the CDC identified Haitian nationality as a risk factor. The

CDC later retracted that statement, but that did not help the 27 percent of Haitian Americans who had lost their jobs. For an insightful analysis of AIDS among Haitians, which frames local experiences of illness in terms of the larger political economy of Haitian-U.S. relations and which includes a reading of conspiracy theories using a "hermeneutic of generosity," see Farmer 1992.

6. Copal is a tree resin used by the Mayans as incense.

CHAPTER 4

1. I met two soldiers from the Belize Defense Forces in a bar in the fishing and tourist village of Placencia. They had just gotten back from military training in Panama City. They were there in the period between the failed coup attempt against General Noriega and the U.S. invasion. They thought it was a giant party! Lines of girls waited on the clipped greensward along which the canal zone's military bases were arrayed. The girls just waited for the soldiers to pick them out and have them for a dollar. You just signed one in at the gate of your post. Beer cost sixty cents a bottle, ten cents a draft. The soldiers were drunk and happy.

2. For the year 1987, the last year before 1990 that these figures were documented, the immigration department reported 310,292 civilians arriving in Belize, which itself boasted a population of only about 170,000. The arrivals include 197,731 returning Belizean residents; 96,747 tourists; 6,443 business and official visitors; and 9,371 travellers passing through between different countries. These figures exclude counts from the entry points of PG and Dangriga (Belize Government 1988, 96).

3. An international advisory group called the Civil-Military Alliance was established in 1996 to begin to deal with the issues I discuss here. For the English version of their newsletter write to 4 West Wheelock Street, Hanover, NH 03755.

4. Compare this to the wages of a sawmill employee's wife who cooks for four men, nine hours a day, six days a week for $78 Bz a week (= $39 US).

5. For simplicity's sake I focus exclusively on HIV here; however, it is important to remember that there are other sexually transmissible viruses, such as hepatitis B and C that, although not fatal, cannot be cured. In addition, symptoms from other STDs, such as ulcerated tissue, facilitate HIV transmission.

6. There has been substantial cross-cultural confirmation regarding the way in which prostitutes mark the distinction between professional and personal sexual contacts, such as not kissing johns and not using condoms with intimate partners; for North American examples, see Jackson et al. 1992; Shedlin and Oliver 1993.

7. Reported cases from gonococcal infection were listed as the third most frequent disease in the nation for 1986–1987 (Belize Government 1988, 53).

8. In a video entitled *AIDS in Belize,* produced in Belize City by Pollard, Woods, and Krohn, the narrator calls sex the national pastime, part of the tropical take-it-easy-and-enjoy-it national identity.

9. The report was presented in Belize at USAID in June 1990 and at the fourth annual studies on Belize conference in October 1990 sponsored by the Society for the Promotion of Education and Research (SPEAR). In response to public questioning at the second event, the National AIDS Coordinator, my co-panelist, presented a revised estimation of ninety-five HIV/AIDS cases, including twenty women citizens, two children, nine immigrants, one refugee, four full-blown cases of AIDS, and twenty-five deaths.

10. The Anglo-Guatemalan dispute was resolved not long after these events. In 1991, the president of Guatemala finally recognized the independence and sovereignty of its nieghbor (Kerns 1997). The British pulled most of its army out by about 1993, and the United States has increased its military presence (Rick Wilk, personal communication, Sept. 16, 1997).

CHAPTER 6

1. Derrida (1993, 10) explains why the humble task of tracing the lay of the land is important: "The responsibilities which anyone (and first and foremost the 'decision maker'—the legislator, educator, citizen in general, etc.) should accept in such an emergency are only all the more serious, difficult and ineluctable. Depending on circumstances (tirelessly analyzed, whether macroscopically or microscopically) a discourse of 'prohibition' can be justified *just as well or just as badly as* a discourse of liberalization. A repressive practice (in all its brutal or sophisticated, punitive or reeducational forms) can be justified just as well or just as badly as a permissive practice (with all its ruses). As one can never fully explicate neither one nor the other of these practices, so one can never absolutely condemn either of them. In an emergency this can only lead to equivocations, negotiations, and unstable compromises. And in any given, progressively evolving situation, these will need to be guided by a concern for the singularity of each individual experience and by a socio-political analysis that is at once as broadly and as finely tuned as possible, I say this not to avoid the question, no more than I do to argue for relativism or opportunism; rather, I would simply describe the lay of the land on which such decisions ought to be made, though the ultimate extent and boundaries of the problem remain unanalyzed and unthought."

2. And just so readers know how far the health agenda was pushed back by

drug war ideology, I tell you that, at the time, project staff were relieved when Jesse Helms's proposed legislation to ban *bleach* distribution to federally funded AIDS prevention programs was not passed. For a recent review of the legal status and activities of needle exchange programs see (CDC 1997).

3. Angel dust, also known as PCP, is a synthetic hallucinogen. MDA is the longer-acting and stronger version of the synthetic stimulant MDMA (= XTC, Ecstasy).

CHAPTER 7

1. Determining whether or not someone is a prostitute is not a particularly useful way of approaching AIDS prevention: It is the pattern of action, not identity, that determines the risk of infection. Indeed, if identity becomes more important than behavior, it can increase risk, as illustrated by the case of Belizean women who work the limeys in the bars. Because they don't want to be stigmatized by the label of prostitution, they carry out the same kinds of sexual behaviors as professional prostitutes but call it something else. For a revealing analysis of the difficulties inherent in using the prostitute label, see Hammar 1996, and for an analysis of the "gendered enclosures" that the prostitute label creates, see Nencel 1997.

2. See Connors (1995), for an analysis of the forms of dissent among injecting drug users.

3. All reused needles serve as viable facilitators of HIV transmission, not just those that carry illegal substances. There is a theory that AIDS was systematically spread in Africa along with the smallpox vaccine. The molecular structure of the smallpox virus seems to be especially conducive to carrying HIV. In his analysis of Black Liberation as a source of counterknowledge, Fiske (1994, 191–216) quotes Zears Miles on Black Liberation Radio uncovering WHO data in support of the theory. The theory has been generally ignored; the widespread imputation of malice on the part of the humanitarian agents of Western medicine would be disastrous.

4. The image of women drug users as passive victims is a popular stereotype matched only by its opposite, the "bad girl." Generally speaking, more men than women choose injection as a mode of drug administration. However, women who are injectors are also harder to find; a larger share of child care responsibilities tend to keep them at home; in some cases, women drug users on the street may be subject to a greater degree of police harassment than men drug users and dealers (Maher 1997, 218). For a review of feminist attempts to set an agenda on women, drug use, and AIDS prevention, see Henderson 1994.

5. Personal communication, Wendell Johnson, Nov. 1995.

CHAPTER 8

1. Anderson's song was released in 1989, two years after Wim Wenders released his film *Wings of Desire,* which took place in Berlin when it was still divided by the wall. The song is based on Walter Benjamin's (1969, 257–58) interpretation of Paul Klee's painting *Angelus Novus.* Locke (1991) analyzes the semiotic interconnections among these works.

CHAPTER 9

1. From the poem, "Down and Out" (in Felleman 1936, 182–84).

2. Even now that all blood products are screened for HIV, transfusion-associated infection is still occurring. Since 1985, an estimated 3,000 people have been infected through blood products in the U.S. (Chapman 1994). The risks are higher in developing countries. For international review of blood supply regulation see Salbu 1996.

3. The quote and summary of events is from a newspaper account (Gregory 1993) and from the records of the Lexington-Fayette County Urban Police Department (post-arrest complaint, case #93–16978, ORI KY0340200, Mar. 27, 1993).

4. Lexington, Kentucky, hosts several Mexican-owned businesses and a large population of migrants who work the tobacco fields.

5. Kathleen Daly (1992) tackles the problem of how feminist criminologists can represent women lawbreakers without overemphasizing their victimhood.

6. The following summary is based on newspaper articles (Campbell 1994; Bennett 1996) and Fayette District Court records (CCN2516666 and 2516667, offense date Jan. 14, 1994).

7. The following summary is based on MacFarquhar 1995.

8. There is a sad and telling rumor on the streets of New York City that some poor people desperate for housing, food, and medical care have purposefully infected themselves so that they could become eligible for benefits (Michele Shedlin, personal communication, May 1997).

9. Research shows that HIV-positive women are likely to be abused when they or others tell their male partners of their infection (e.g., North and Rothenberg 1993).

10. For example, once I interviewed a Mexican man in Chicago. Like the other Mexicans he knew in the city, he left his loved ones in Mexico. He and his compatriots occasionally went out drinking and had sex with prostitutes. He was living with an injector, but didn't know it. His partner had told project staff that she injected drugs, but we nevertheless could inform him in only the most gen-

eralized way about risks associated with needle use. His partner would have to take it upon herself to clarify the close-to-home nature of his risk.

11. Cuban filmmakers Ivan Arocha and David Hernandez produced the film, which was screened at the 1993 annual meetings of the American Anthropological Association. Some time after *Beyond Outcasts* was made, the Cuban public health officials abandoned the mandatory quarantine strategy. They switched to an open approach, wherein anyone who is HIV-infected could choose to come reside in sanitoria and receive free medicine, room, and board. For a discussion of how Cuban AIDS care developed in response to the changing epidemic, see Santana 1997.

12. This summary is based on Malcomson 1994 and Ina Rosa 1995. The Rockers are also known as the *Roqueros, Los Injectados,* Freekiss (sounds like Freakies), and Rebels Without A Cause.

CHAPTER 10

1. China invaded Tibet in the late 1950s. Rinpoche fled, disrobed, and was provided with the means to study art and philosophy at Oxford before settling in Boulder to establish Vajradhatu, representing the Kagyu school, one of the four schools of Tibetan Buddhism.

2. The editor was Rick Fields, author of *Carrying Water, Chopping Wood* and *The Swans Come to the Lake,* about Buddhism in North America.

3. The state of Colorado does not now (1997), and did not then, have any laws concerning the intentional or knowing transmission of HIV by persons other than HIV-positive prostitutes or their clients.

However, all states that apply for funds under the Ryan White Comprehensive AIDS Resources Emergency Act of 1990 are required to warrant that their criminal statutes could prosecute a person who has been informed of his or her HIV infection and who either donates blood, semen, or breast milk; engages in sexual activity; or shares hypodermic needles with intent to expose others to HIV. The act does not require the enactment of HIV-specific statutes, only that a state have adequate criminal statues to prosecute such conduct (Report of the Presidential Commission on the Human Immunodeficiency Virus Epidemic 1988, 130, cited in Tierney 1992).

CHAPTER 11

1. The following summary is based on Blanchfield's 1994 newspaper account.

2. The following summary is based on six newspaper accounts: Bain 1993; Bergman and Johnson 1995; Dambrofsky 1995a, 1995b, 1995c; and Feschuk 1995.

CHAPTER 12

1. The data in this chapter were collected as part of the larger survey of intentional HIV transmission cases in the United States between 1986 and 1996. A comprehensive Lexis-Nexis search was combined with newspaper articles and television shows that I happened to come across or that friends and family sent. Ted Swedenburg (personal communication, Nov. 1992) told me the Egyptian film example. Leon Pettiway (personal communication, Dec. 1996) told me the Caribbean example.

Structural analysis of texts derives from the methods of Propp 1958; Lévi-Strauss 1967; and Jameson 1981. I use myself as experimental subject to produce hypotheses regarding the relationship between narrative structure and audience effects.

2. The word "casual" belies the very intense emotions that often accompany ephemeral sexual relationships.

3. When a representative of the conservative Heritage Foundation in Washington, D.C., one William Donohue, came on *Larry King Live* (Cable News Network 1992, 5–6) to argue for tougher criminal laws against intentional HIV transmission, he provided this example to support his perspective: "He [one of his students] tells me of a case of a girl whom he knows who went on spring break down to Florida and had a good time, and she had sex with some young fellow. And on the way coming back in the plane, she opens up a present from him in the midst of the other girls. She opens up the box, and there's a little gold coffin. And inside the coffin there's a little note which says, 'I've got aids [*sic*], and you've got it now, too.' She tested positive for aids [*sic*]."

4. This show was aired on Channel 6, WRTV, on the evening of March 28, 1995.

5. The detectives essentially proceed to do contact tracing, a basic prevention and treatment procedure for tracking down syphilis and gonorrhea cases. With some exceptions, contract tracing is not used to track AIDS in the United States because of confidentiality laws.

6. The program aired on the Discovery channel on the evening of May 19, 1996.

7. *State of Oregon, Respondent, v. Timothy Alan Hinkhouse, Appellant* CA A84175.

8. Nor does the medical profession provide any backup. In her critique of the "sacred cow" of total confidentiality, Elinor Burkett (1995, 207) explains that some states give physicians permission to inform spouses, or ask the city's partner-notification officer to do so, if they have clear reason to believe that the sero-

positive spouse will not do so. But violations of confidentiality carry fines of up to five thousand dollars, and few physicians will risk overstepping bounds. In New York, not one physican had ever referred a name to the contact-tracing office by 1993.

9. Note that this sample represents only a fraction of the cases that have occurred or are in process. There is no systematic documentation of these cases. Most never appear in national media or get picked up on Nexis data bases. For the most part, they get picked up in the Lexis legal data bases and then only after the appeals process and only if a judge decides to write up the decision. The delays and haphazardness of documentation make a comprehensive case search impossible. However, given the relative rarity of cases, it would seem that there is a disproportionate level of legislative action.

10. As Rosenberg (1988, 28–29) explains, different frames of reference are used to interpret scientific knowledge. Accurate descriptions of the natural world often become distorted as they inform moral and legal discourses. Not unlike public reactions to cholera a century and a half ago, immunologists' suggestions that AIDS may grow out of successive assaults on the immune system may be transcoded to mean that people with AIDS have predisposed themselves. When epidemiologists correlate the incidence of AIDS with numbers of sexual contacts, speaking in terms of likelihoods, nonscientists may start thinking in terms of individual guilt and deserved punishment.

/ Bibliography

Aiken, Jane, and Michael Musheno. 1994. Why have-nots win the HIV litigation arena: Socio-legal dynamics of extreme cases. *Law and Policy* 16(3): 267–98.

Alexander, Priscilla. 1996. Bathhouses and brothels: Symbolic sites in discourse and practice. In *Policing Public Sex: Queer Politics and the Future of AIDS Activism,* Dangerous Bedfellows, eds., 221–50. Boston: South End Press.

Altman, Lawrence. 1997. Case of H.I.V. transmission is first to be linked to kiss: Blood, not saliva, is believed to be cause. *New York Times,* July 10, p. A14.

Andersen, Ellen. 1994. Bad blood: The story of hemophilia and AIDS. Paper presented at the annual meetings of the Law and Society Association, June, Phoenix.

Arendt, Hannah. 1964. *Eichmann in Jerusalem.* New York: Viking Press.

Associated Press. 1990. Osel Tendzin, 47, head of Tibetan Buddhists, dies. *New York Times,* Aug. 28, p. D22.

———. 1993. Texas girls say they had sex with an HIV-infected male to get into gang. *Baltimore Sun,* Apr. 27, p. A7.

———. 1996. Race with death. *Winnipeg Sun,* Mar. 25, p. 38.

———. 1997. Tests: Cunanan HIV negative. *Herald-Times,* Aug. 2, p. A6.

Bain, Jennifer. 1993. Early Boland hearing. *Edmonton Sun,* Aug. 18, p. 4.

Barthes, Roland. 1972. *Mythologies.* New York: Hill and Wang.

Baudrillard, Jean. 1993. *The Transparency of Evil: Essays on Extreme Phenomena.* Translated by James Benedict. New York: Verso.

Belize Government. 1988. *Abstract of Statistics.* Belize City.

Belize Ministry of Health. 1990. World AIDS day. *Community Health News* No. 6 (Nov.–Dec.), p. 1. Edited by Jaqui Roe, Health Education Bureau (HECOBAB), Belize City.

Benjamin, Walter. 1969. *Illuminations.* New York: Schocken.

Bennett, Brian. 1996. Foster back in Fayette after troubled stays in other lockups. *Lexington Herald-Leader,* Nov. 20, pp. A1, A5.

Bergman, Beth. 1988. AIDS, prostitution, and the use of historical stereotypes to legislate sexuality. *John Marshall Law Review* 21: 777–830.

Bergman, Brian, and Bart Johnson. 1995. A fatal attraction? *Maclean's*, May 15, p. 19.

Best, Joel. 1991. Bad guys and random violence: Folklore and media constructions of contemporary deviants. *Contemporary Legend* 1: 107–21.

Blanchfield, Mike. 1994. Life sentence for survivor of "pact in crime." *Edmonton Journal*, June 22, p. A3.

Bond, George, John Kreniske, Ida Susser, and Joan Vincent. 1997. *AIDS in Africa and the Caribbean*. Boulder, Colo.: Westview Press.

Breitbart, Vicki, Wendy Chavkin, and Paul Wise. 1994. The accessibility of drug treatment for pregnant women: A survey of programs in five cities. *American Journal of Public Health* 84(10):1658–61.

Brummelhuis, Han ten, and Gilbert Herdt, eds. 1995. *Culture and Sexual Risk: Anthropological Perspectives*. New York: Gordon and Breach.

Burkett, Elinor. 1995. *The Gravest Show on Earth: America in the Age of AIDS*. Boston: Houghton Mifflin.

Cable News Network (CNN). 1992. Sex and aids—Assault with a deadly weapon? *Larry King Live*, May 13 (transcript).

Calwood, June. 1995. *Trial Without End: A Shocking Story of Women and AIDS*. Toronto: Alfred A. Knopf Canada.

Campbell, Robert. 1994. Foster accuses inmate of trying to giver her HIV. *Lexington Herald-Leader*, Feb. 3, p. B3.

Cantwell, Alan. 1988. *AIDS and the Doctors of Death: An Inquiry into the Origin of the AIDS Epidemic*. San Francisco: Aries Rising.

———. 1993. *Queer Blood: The Secret AIDS Genocide Plot*. San Francisco: Aries Rising.

Carpignano, Paolo, Robin Andersen, Stanley Aronowitz, and William DiFazio. 1993. Chatter in the age of electronic reproduction: Talk television and the "Public Mind." In *The Phantom Public Sphere*, ed. Bruce Robbins for the Social Text Collective, 93–120. Minneapolis: University of Minnesota Press.

CBS News. 1996. *60 Minutes*. November 10, Transcript 29 (9). New Jersey: Burrelle's Transcripts.

Centers for Disease Control and Prevention (CDC). 1981. "Pneumocystis" pneumonia—Los Angeles. *Morbidity and Mortality: Weekly Report* 30(21): 250–52.

———. 1997. Update: Syringe-exchange programs in the United States, 1996. *Morbidity and Mortality: Weekly Report* 46(24):565–74.

Chapman, Michael. 1994. How safe is the blood supply? *Consumers' Report,* April, pp. 10, 14, 15.

Colson, Charles, and Ellen Vaughn. 1995. *Gideon's Torch.* Dallas: Word.

Cook, Timothy, and David Colby. 1992. The mass-mediated epidemic: The politics of AIDS on the nightly network news. In *AIDS: The Making of a Chronic Disease,* Elizabeth Fee and Daniel Fox, eds., 84–122. Berkeley: University of California Press.

Connors, Margaret. 1995. The politics of marginalization: The appropriation of AIDS prevention messages among injection drug users. *Culture, Medicine and Psychiatry* 19:425–52.

———. 1996. Sex, drugs, and structural violence. In *Women, Poverty, and AIDS: Sex, Drugs, and Structural Violence,* Farmer, Connors, and Simmons, eds., 91–123.

Crimp, Douglas. 1987. How to have promiscuity in an epidemic. *AIDS: Cultural Analysis, Cultural Activism.* Special issue edited by Douglas Crimp. Oct. 43:237–71.

Cuomo, Chris. 1996. War is not just an event: Reflections on the significance of everyday violence. *Hypatia* 11(4):30–45.

Curtis, Tom. 1992. The Origin of AIDS. *Rolling Stone,* Mar. 19, p. 56.

Dalton, Harlon. 1993. Criminal law. In *AIDS Law Today: A New Guide for the Public,* Scott Burris, Harlon Dalton, Judith Leonie Miller, and the Yale AIDS Law Project, eds., 242–62. New Haven, Conn.: Yale University Press.

Daly, Kathleen. 1992. Women's pathways to felony court: Feminist theories of lawbreaking and problems of representation. *Southern California Review of Law and Women's Studies* 2(1):11–52.

Dambrofsky, Gwen. 1995a. Witness doubted HIV threat. *Winnipeg Free Press,* May 11, p. A9.

———. 1995b. Expert witness in Tan trial delivers lecture on HIV. *Winnipeg Free Press,* May 13. p. A5

———. 1995c. "Fairy Godfather" feared disgrace, Tan trial told. *Winnipeg Free Press,* May 17, p. A3.

Dangerous Bedfellows (Ephen Colter, Wayne Hoffman, Eva Pendleton, Alison Redick, David Serlin), eds. 1996. *Policing Public Sex: Queer Politics and the Future of AIDS Activism.* Boston: South End Press.

Derrida, Jacques. 1993. The rhetoric of drugs: An interview. Special issue "On Addiction." *Differences* 5:1–25.

Donahue, Phil. 1991. People who intentionally spread the AIDS virus. *Donahue. Show* 1227-91. Transcript 3368. New York: Multimedia Entertainment.

Dotson, Jason. 1977. The female toast teller. Unpublished manuscript.

Douceron, Hervé, Lionel Deforges, Romain Gherardi, Alain Sobel, and Patrick Chariot. 1993. Long-lasting postmortem viability of human immunodeficiency virus: A potential risk in forensic medicine practice. *Forensic Science International* 60(1–2): 61–66.

Drake, St. Clair, and Horace Cayton. 1970. *Black Metropolis: A Study of Negro Life in a Northern City.* New York: Harcourt, Brace and World.

Elliot, Richard. 1997. *Criminal Law and HIV/AIDS: Final Report.* Montreal: Canadian HIV/AIDS Legal Network and the Canadian AIDS Society.

Elshtain, Jean Bethke. 1987. *Women and War.* New York: Basic Books, 166–67.

Enloe, Cynthia. 1989. *Bananas, Beaches, and Bases: Making Feminist Sense of International Politics.* Berkeley: University of California Press.

Erni, John Nguyet. 1994. *Unstable Frontiers: Technomedicine and the Cultural Politics of "Curing" AIDS.* Minneapolis: University of Minnesota Press.

Falk Moore, Sally. 1973. Law and social change: The semi-autonomous social field as an appropriate subject of study. *Law and Society Review* 7(4): 719–46.

Farmer, Paul. 1992. *AIDS and Accusation: Haiti and the Geography of Blame.* Berkeley: University of California Press.

Farmer, Paul, Margaret Connors, and Janie Simmons, eds. 1996. *Women, Poverty, and AIDS: Sex, Drugs, and Structural Violence.* Monroe, Maine: Common Courage Press.

Farmer, Paul, Shirley Lindenbaum, and Mary-Jo Delvecchio Good, eds. 1993. Women, Poverty, and AIDS. Special Issue of *Culture, Medicine and Psychiatry* 17(4): 387–97.

Featherstone, Mike. 1995. *Undoing Culture: Globalization, Postmodernism and Identity.* Thousand Oaks, Calif.: Sage.

Feldman, Douglas. 1990. *Culture and AIDS.* New York: Praeger.

Felleman, Hazel. 1936. *The Best Loved Poems of the American People.* Garden City, N.Y.: Doubleday.

Fernando, M. Daniel. 1993. *AIDS and Intravenous Drug Use: The Influence of Morality, Politics, Social Science, and Race in the Making of a Tragedy.* Westport, Conn.: Praeger.

Ferrell, Jeff. 1996. *Crimes of Style: Urban Graffiti and the Politics of Criminality.* Boston: Northeastern University Press.

Feschuk, Scott. Photographer's AIDS called result of lifestyle, not Tan. *Globe and Mail,* May 20, p. A4.

Field, Martha, and Kathleen Sullivan. 1987. AIDS and the criminal law. *Law, Medicine, and Health Care* 15(1–2): 46–60.

Fine, Gary. 1992. *Manufacturing Tales: Sex and Money in Contemporary Legends.* Knoxville: University of Tennessee.

Fiske, John. 1994. *Media Matters: Everyday Culture and Political Change.* Minneapolis: University of Minnesota Press.

Frankenburg, Ronald. 1995. Learning from AIDS: The future of anthropology. In *The Future of Anthropology: Its Relevance to the Contemporary World,* Akbar Ahmed and Cris Shore, eds., 110–33. London: Athlone Press.

Glick-Schiller, Nina. 1992. What's wrong with this picture? The hegemonic construction of culture in AIDS research in the United States. *Medical Anthropology Quarterly* 6: 237–54.

Goldstein, Diane. 1992. Welcome to the mainland, welcome to the world of AIDS: Cultural viability, localization and contemporary legend. *Contemporary Legend* 2: 23–40.

Gordon, Diana. 1990. *The Justice Juggernaut: Fighting Street Crime, Controlling Citizens.* New Brunswick, N.J.: Rutgers University Press.

Gostin, Lawrence. 1996. *The AIDS Litigation Project: A Look at HIV/AIDS in the Courts of the 1990s.* Washington, D.C.: Kaiser Family Foundation.

Gregory, Eric. 1993. Ex-Lexington prostitute says she tried to transmit HIV. *Lexington Herald-Leader,* October 2, pp. A1, A8.

Greene, Warner. 1993. AIDS and the immune system. *Scientific American* 269(3): 99–105.

Guillot Hurtubise, Bruno. 1996. 30 months imprisonment for syringe attack. *Canadian HIV/AIDS Policy and Law Newsletter* 1(1). On the Internet: *www.juris.uqam.ca/resdsida/VOLNO1/ENGL1-1/106.htm.*

Hall, Stuart. 1993. Culture, Community, Nation *Cultural Studies* 7(3): 349–63.

Hammar, Lawrence. 1996. Bad canoes and *bafalo:* The political economy of sex on Daru Island, Western Province, Papua New Guinea. *Genders* 23: 212–43.

Hannaham, James. 1996. Positively Criminal. *Out.* May, 72–73.

Haraway, Donna. 1991. *Simians, Cyborgs, and Women: The Reinvention of Nature.* New York: Routledge.

Hebdige, Dick. 1988. *Subculture: The Meaning of Style.* New York: Routledge.

Henderson, Sheila. 1994. Time for a makeover? Women and drugs in the contexts of AIDS. In *AIDS: Setting a Feminist Agenda,* Lesley Doyal, Jennie Naidoo, and Tamsin Wilton, eds., 183–96. Bristol, Pa.: Taylor and Francis.

Herdt, Gilbert, and Shirley Lindenbaum. 1992. *The Time of AIDS: Social Analysis, Theory and Method.* Newbury Park, Calif.: Sage.

Ina Rosa, Maria. 1995. National Public Radio, Aug. 8, evening news.

Jackson, Lois, Alexandra Highcrest, and Randall Coates. 1992. Varied potential risks of HIV infection among prostitutes. *Social Science and Medicine* 35(3): 281–86.

Jameson, Fredric. 1981. *The Political Unconscious: Narrative as a Socially Symbolic Act.* Ithaca, N.Y.: Cornell University Press.

———. 1994. *Postmodernism, or, the Cultural Logic of Late Capitalism.* Durham, N.C.: Duke University Press.

Johnson, Wendell. 1994. *"Carrying a Stick": Homelessness Among African American Injecting Drug Users in Chicago.* Ph.D. dissertation. Northwestern University.

Joint United Nations Programme on HIV/AIDS. 1996. The HIV/AIDS situation in mid-1996: Global and regional highlights. *UNAIDS Fact Sheet,* July 1.

Kalichman, Seth, J. Greenberg, and G. G. Abel. 1997. HIV seropositive men who engage in high risk sexual behavior: Psychological characteristics and implications for prevention. *AIDS Care* 9(4): 441–50.

Kane, Stephanie. 1993. Race, sex work, and ethnographic representation, or, what to do about Loki's toast. *Canadian Folklore canadien* 15(1): 109–17.

———. 1994. *The Phantom Gringo Boat: Shamanic Discourse and Development in Panama.* Washington, D.C.: Smithsonian.

Kane, Stephanie, and Theresa Mason. 1992. "IV drug users" and "sex partners": The limits of epidemiological categories and the ethnography of risk. In *Social Analysis in the Time of AIDS: Theory, Method, and Action.* Herdt and Lindenbaum, eds., 199–224.

Kerns, Virginia. 1997. *Women and the Ancestors: Black Carib Kinship and Ritual.* 2d ed. Urbana: University of Illinois Press.

Leonard, Arthur. 1993. *Sexuality and the Law: An Encyclopedia of Major Legal Cases.* New York: Garland.

Lévi-Strauss, Claude. 1967. *Structural Anthropology.* Garden City, N.Y.: Doubleday.

Locke, Liz. 1991. Strange Angels: Recontextualizing Walter Benjamin and Laurie Anderson. Unpublished manuscript.

MacFarquhar, Neil. 1995. Downward spiral of troubled life. *New York Times,* June 27, pp. B1, B4.

MacQueen, Kathleen. 1994. The epidemiology of HIV transmission: Trends, structure and dynamics. *Annual Review of Anthropology* 23: 509–26.

Maher, Lisa. 1997. *Sexed Work: Gender, Race, and Resistance in a Brooklyn Drug Market.* New York: Oxford University Press.

Malcomson, Scott. 1994. Socialism or death? *The New York Times Magazine,* September 25, pp. 44–50.

Marcus, George. 1995. Ethnography in/of the world system: The emergence of multi-sited ethnography, *Annual Review of Anthropology* 24:95–117.

Martin, Emily. 1994. *Flexible Bodies: Tracking Immunity in American Culture from the Days of Polio to the Age of AIDS.* Boston: Beacon Press.

Miller, William. 1993. *Humiliation: And Other Essays on Honor, Social Discomfort, and Violence.* Ithaca: Cornell University Press.

Minkowitz, Donna. 1996. Wrath-of-God best sellers. *The Nation* 262(7):25–28.

National Commission on AIDS. 1992. *The Challenge of HIV/AIDS in Communities of Color.* Washington, D.C.

Nencel, Lorraine. 1997. *Casting Identities, Gendered Enclosures: Women who Prostitute in Lima, Peru.* Ph.D. dissertation. Universiteit van Amsterdam.

Niedringhaus, Landon. 1990. *The Public Health Implications of Medical Waste: A Report to Congress.* Atlanta: U.S. Dept. of Health and Human Services.

North, Richard and Karen Rothenberg. 1993. Partner notification and the threat of domestic violence against women with HIV infection. *New England Journal of Medicine* 329(16):1194–96.

Padian, Nancy. 1990. Sexual histories of heterosexual couples with one HIV-infected partner. *American Journal of Public Health* 80:990–91.

Patterson, David. 1995. *HIV: Public Health, Criminal Law and the Process of Policy Development.* Master's thesis. Faculty of Law, McGill University.

Presidential Commission on the Human Immunodeficiency Virus Epidemic. 1988. *Report.* Washington, D.C.

Propp, Vladimir. 1958. *Morphology of the Folktale.* The Hague: Mouton.

Roberts, Dorothy. 1995. Motherhood and crime. *Social Text* 42:99–123.

Ronell, Avital. 1992. *Crack Wars: Literature Addiction Mania.* Lincoln: University of Nebraska Press.

Rosenberg, Charles. 1988. Disease and social order in America: Perceptions and expectations. In *AIDS: The Burdens of History,* Elizabeth Fee and Daniel Fox, eds., 12–32. Berkeley: University of California Press.

Royce, Rachel, Arlene Seña, Willard Cates, and Myron Cohen. 1997. Sexual transmission of HIV. *New England Journal of Medicine* 336(15):1072–78.

Salbu, Steven. 1996. AIDS and the blood supply: An analysis of law, regulation, and public policy. *Washington University Law Quarterly* 74 (4):913–80.

Santana, Sarah. 1997. AIDS prevention, treatment, and care in Cuba. In *AIDS in*

Africa and the Caribbean, Bond, Kreniske, Susser, and Vincent, eds., 65–84.

Scott, Peter Dale, and Jonathan Marshall. 1991. *Cocaine Politics: Drugs, Armies, and the CIA in Central America.* Berkeley: University of California Press.

Shedlin, Michele, and Denise Oliver. 1993. Prostitution and HIV risk behavior. In *Advances in Population: Psychosocial Perspectives,* Lawrence Severy, ed. Vol. 1:157–72. Philadelphia: Jessica Kingsley Publishers.

Shilts, Randy. 1987. *And the Band Played On: Politics, People, and the AIDS Epidemic.* New York: St. Martin's Press.

Singer, Linda. 1993. *Erotic Welfare: Sexual Theory and Politics in the Age of Epidemics.* New York: Routledge.

Singer, Merrill. 1998. *The Political Economy of AIDS.* Amityville, N.Y.: Baywood Publishing Co.

Smart, Carol. 1995. *Law, Crime and Sexuality: Essays in Feminism.* Thousand Oaks, Calif.: Sage.

Sobo, Elisa. 1995. *Choosing Safe Sex: AIDS-Risk Denial Among Disadvantaged Women.* Philadelphia: University of Pennsylvania Press.

Stall, Ron, Suzanne Heurtin-Roberts, Leon McKusick, Colleen Hoff, and Sylvia Wanner Lang. 1990. Sexual risk for HIV transmission among singles-bar patrons in San Francisco. *Medical Anthropology Quarterly* 4(1):115–28.

Sterk-Elifson, Claire. 1993. Outreach among drug users: Combining the role of ethnographic field assistant and health educator. *Human Organization* 52(2):162–68.

Sullivan, Kathleen, and Martha Field. 1988. AIDS and the coercive power of the state. *Harvard Civil Rights-Civil Liberties Law Review* 23:139–97.

Taussig, Michael. 1997. *The Magic of the State.* New York: Routledge.

Tierney, Thomas. 1992. Criminalizing the sexual transmission of HIV: An international analysis. *Hastings International and Comparative Law Review* 15: 475–513.

U.S. Department of Justice. 1996. Prosecutors in State Courts, 1994. *Bureau of Justice Statistics Bulletin* (NCJ-151656). Washington, D.C.

———. 1997. Lifetime likelihood of going to state or federal prison. Bureau of Justice Statistics Special Report (NCJ-160092). Washington, D.C.

Watney, Simon. 1994. *Practices of Freedom: Selected Writings on HIV/AIDS.* Durham, N.C.: Duke University Press.

Webber, David. 1997. *AIDS and the Law.* 3d ed. Colorado Springs, Colo.: Wiley Law.

Wiebel, Wayne, Thomas Lampinen, Douglas Ward-Chene and Barbara Stevko

1990. HIV-1 Seroconversion in a cohort of street intravenous drug users in Chicago. Poster presented at the Sixth International Conference on AIDS, San Francisco, June.

Williams, Patricia. 1991. *The Alchemy of Race and Rights: Diary of a Law Professor.* Cambridge: Harvard University Press.

Williams, Raymond. 1961. *The Long Revolution.* Harmondsworth: Penguin.

————. 1977. *Marxism and Literature.* New York: Oxford.

World Health Organization (WHO). 1991. *Weekly Epidemiological Record* 67(3):9.

————. 1994. *Weekly Epidemiological Record* 69(37):274.

————. 1997. *Weekly Epidemiological Record* 72(27):197.

Zink, Karin. 1992. Love v. Superior Court: Mandatory AIDS testing and prostitution. *Golden Gate University Law Review* 22:795–817.

/ Index

Names that have been changed by the author for the purposes of preserving anonymity appear in quotation marks. Historically accurate names, including pseudonyms in common usage, are not so marked.